CREATIVE AROMATHERAPY

These immemorial essences fill the r
with purple haze and auroral mist, c
impalpable visions of ancient things.

MARY WEBB

CHRISTINE WILDWOOD is an experienced aromatherapist and Bach Flower practitioner. As well as writing a number of magazine articles on health-related subjects, she is the author of several books, including *Holistic Aromatherapy*. She lives in South Wales and runs a holistic health practice from her home.

Creative
Aromatherapy

CHRISTINE WILDWOOD

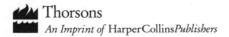
Thorsons
An Imprint of HarperCollins*Publishers*

Thorsons
An Imprint of HarperCollins*Publishers*
77—85 Fulham Palace Road
Hammersmith, London W6 8JB
1160 Battery Street
San Francisco, California 94111—1213

Published by Thorsons 1993
10 9 8 7 6 5 4 3 2 1

A catalogue record for this book
is available from the British Library

ISBN 0 7225 2826 4

Typeset by Harper Phototypesetters Limited,
Northampton, England
Printed in Great Britain by
Woolnough Bookbinding, Irthlingborough, Northants

Contents

Introduction   7

1 Aroma   9
2 The Essence of the Art   19
3 Essential Oil Profiles   27
4 Aromatherapy Techniques   45
5 The Alchemist's Larder   77
6 Apprenticed to Alchemy   84
7 Psychic Scents   106
8 Ambience in the Making   121
9 Other Dimensions   137

Further Reading   153
Appendix: Essential Oil Suppliers   154
Therapeutic Index   156
General Index   158

Acknowledgements

Thank you, Peter and Andrew, for initiating me into the mysteries of word processing. And also to you, Frank, for rescuing the alchemist's apprentice from limbo just when I thought he'd gone forever! Rose, a very warm thank you for your loyal friendship and your lovely words.

And to you, Mum and Dad, for being so special.

Finally, thanks to Jane Graham-Maw of Thorsons for the initial inspiration: it has been a joy to write.

Introduction

Within the span of a decade, aromatherapy has emerged from the mists of relative obscurity into the sunshine of popular awareness. Just why it should have captured the imagination on such a grand scale is not too difficult to understand. Apart from the remarkable healing properties of plant essences, or 'essential oils' as they are commonly called, the practice of aromatherapy appeals to our aesthetic nature. Moreover, it is one of the few healing arts which could be described as 'creative' in an artistic sense. This is because much of the skill of the aromatherapist (or the 'adventurous essential oil user') lies in the ability to concoct wonderful mood-enhancing aromas. This is achieved by blending oils and essences, floral waters and beeswax, and other intriguing bounties born of a fragrant Earth.

Unlike more clinical therapies such as homoeopathy or acupuncture, aromatherapy's healing potential stems from its ability to promote relaxation and to engender a sense of joy or tranquillity in the recipient. In so doing, it creates favourable conditions within body and mind for healing to take place quite naturally.

Aromatherapy combines fragrant oils with massage, thus making full use of our most primitive, yet most highly evolved senses: smell and touch. Add gentle music and a pleasing decor and we also nurture our auditory and visual senses. Above all, aromatherapy embraces the spiritual aspect of our being, for Tender Loving Care is the most potent healing force of all.

Even though massage is the mainstay of the art of aromatherapy, essential oils can be used in a variety of other ways for healing or simply for pleasure — in baths, skin care preparations and as uplifting perfumes, for example. Unfortunately, the art of massage therapy (as practised by pro-fessional aromatherapists) is beyond the scope of this book, whose emphasis is on mixing and blending oils for their psychotherapeutic effects. However, a simplified massage sequence which will serve as a starter is described in Chapter 4. For those wishing to go further, the Further Reading List gives details of books on aromatherapy and massage, and the Appendix lists the addresses of some very good training establishments.

Creative aromatherapy is less about choosing oils to treat specific problems (though this approach is given space), rather it is about exploring our subjective, yet profoundly real responses to the subtleties of aroma. Therefore, no matter whether you are an experienced wayfarer on the fragrant path or one who travels hopefully, this book will guide you deeper into the art of aromatherapy and self-awareness.

My own work in aromatherapy includes the use of the Bach Flower Remedies. These Remedies, which are similar to homoeopathic medicines in that infinitesimal quantities are administered, were discovered in the 1930s by the visionary physician Dr Edward Bach. In this method of healing, certain wild flowers are selected for their special ability to treat the personality and distressing emotions of the sufferer rather than the physical symptoms of their illness. The Flower Remedies (which are now widely available from health shops) are highly compatible with aromatherapy, broadening the psycho-therapeutic effects of the oils. In the final chapter of this book you will find a number of suggestions for incorporating the Flower Remedies into your aromatic concoctions, thus adding another dimension to the alchemy of fragrance.

The purpose of this book is to encourage readers to be free and creative in the art of blending essential oils for therapeutic or aesthetic purposes. Although it has been said that blending aromatics is a skill which requires training and a great deal of practice, I believe it is more to do with enthusiasm combined with imagination and a genuine love of the art. As a matter of interest, the most talented fragrance makers I know tend also to be imaginative cooks. If cooking is not your forté, however, do not despair. With a little guidance and the highest quality essences and vegetable oils, you too can make interesting blends. The secret is simply to let go and enjoy!

Christine Wildwood, August, 1992

1 · Aroma

A Silent Language

It is almost impossible to describe an aroma to someone who has not smelled it before. At best, we can only compare it with other scents, or with textures, sounds and flavours. For instance, it may smell like vanilla fudge, like lemon, wet leaves or camphor. Or, more imaginatively, like a cacophony of nostril-stinging scents, each screaming for attention (the perfume counter at a discount chain store) . . . or like wood dipped in honey and the finest velvet (essence of sandalwood).

Yet aroma has a mute language of its own. Nothing is more evocative. A mere whiff of a certain scent may unexpectedly conjure up memories of first love, perhaps, another, endless summer days by the sea when the sun blazed in a clear blue sky, a third, a childhood visit to the local 'oil shop' whose scrubbed wooden floors, hessian sacks of potatoes, ironmongery and bundles of kindling sticks drenched the air with a comforting earthy scent.

Joy aside, however, it is equally true to say that certain aromas, no matter how pleasing to most people, will evoke distressful memories in one who may associate the odour with some unpleasant experience. I know of one woman, for instance, who cannot abide the scent of rose. It reminds her of an unhappy episode during her schooldays, in particular of the harsh schoolmistress who always smelled of a rose-scented perfume. Another example involves a young man of my acquaintance who suffers occasional panic attacks triggered by the aroma of butterscotch. Strangely, he cannot recall a deeply held association with the aroma, yet it seems likely that something disturbing in this connection must have occurred in his life at some point, possibly during early childhood.

So the effect of aroma upon the mind and emotions is powerful and immediate; yet there is no short-term memory with odour. Hit that elusive switch and you are transported across space-time into the Eternal Now — of memories, feelings and visions. What you experience may appear to be fleeting, but can be experienced over and over again.

In Times Past

As far back in time as any archaeologist can decipher, people have been intrigued by the seemingly magical potency of aroma. Our early ancestors used their highly developed sensory and intuitive powers to single out not only the culinary and medicinal plants, but also, more interestingly, those which gave rise to altered states of consciousness. It was found that when certain aromatic plants and plant resins were burnt as incense, some aromas made people feel relaxed or drowsy while others made them feel uplifted, even euphoric, and the most precious of all gave rise to certain mystical states. These aromatic gifts of the great Earth Mother were burnt only by the priests and priestesses during magico-religious rites or for healing purposes. Since healing and religion were interrelated, the 'smoking' of sick people (often to exorcise evil spirits) became an important aspect of the healer's art.

The ancient Egyptians, however, are generally regarded as the true founders of aromatherapy. They used aromatics for religious ceremonies and embalming, as well as for healing, which included massage, and for cosmetic purposes.

The formulae for many aromatic concoctions were carved into the stone walls of Egyptian temples, allowing us access to some of the most mind-bending preparations. Kyphi, for instance, perhaps the best known of the Egyptian incenses, is a luxurious and heady brew consisting of no less than 16 ingredients, including saffron, cassia, spikenard, cinnamon and juniper. Dioscorides called it a perfume welcome to the gods. Kyphi was always burnt after sunset, not only to ensure the safe return of the Sun God Ra, but also because its effects were soporific and intoxicating.

Then there was Theriaque, another exotic concoction, which was believed to dispel anxiety. Theriaque was composed of between 57 and 96 ingredients (temple recipes vary), which included myrrh, cinnamon, rush, sweet flak, juniper and cassia — and, less aesthetically, serpent skin and spittle!

In ancient China, wealthy households had a special room for childbirth called the artemesia room, where the plant (also known as mugwort) was burned to attract kindred spirits and to bring about a state of joy to both mother and child. More interestingly, the Chinese were also involved with the quest for immortality through the practice of alchemy. An alchemist would burn incense and douse himself with specially prepared perfume before carrying out his experiments. It was believed that the fragrance of plants held magical forces and plant spirits whose power would help in concocting the Elixir of Life.

Throughout the ancient world frankincense resin, extracted from trees grown in southwest Arabia, was traded; and in a spiritual sense was far more precious than gold. For when burnt as incense, it was believed that the aromatic vapour elevated the spirit, linking the human psyche with the powerful energies of the gods.

Incidentally, frankincense is still burnt as incense in Catholic churches, but I wonder how many priests are aware that its clear resinous aroma has the ability to deepen the breathing? As every meditator knows, deep breathing calms the mind, which in turn, relaxes the body, thus creating a state inducive to prayer and meditation. However, there is more to it than this: in 1981 scientists in Germany decided to investigate reports of the so-called 'mind-bending effects' of inhaling the aroma of frankincense. (Altar boys were said to have become emotionally addicted to the substance.) It was found that when frankincense was burned, it produced trahydrocannabinole, a psychoactive substance which is known to expand the subconscious.

Many great thinkers of the past have paid tribute to the power inherent in fragrance, not only to influence mood and to evoke memories, but to facilitate original thought. Montaigne declared that incense and perfume had the power 'to comfort, to quicken, to rouse, and to purify our senses so that we might

11

be apter and readier into contemplation'. And Proust, when he lived in Paris, would travel 100 kilometres to Normandy just to inhale the scent of apple blossom, which he believed gave him direct access to the fount of inspiration. The German dramatist and poet Schiller would wait until the autumn before indulging in his 'fix' of the Tree of Knowledge. He used to keep rotten apples in the drawer of his desk and inhale their pungent aroma whenever he needed to find the right word or phrase. He was certainly on to something. Researchers at Yale University in the USA have discovered that the aroma of apples and cinnamon has a powerful 'grounding' or stabilizing effect on some people, especially those suffering from nervous anxiety. The aroma has even been known to lower high blood pressure and to stave off panic attacks. But how is this possible?

The Sense of Smell

The area of the brain associated with smell (the olfactory centre) is very closely connected with the limbic portion of the brain, which is concerned with our basic drives such as hunger, thirst and sex drive, and also our most subtle responses such as emotion, memory, creativity and intuition. The olfactory area also connects with the hypothalamus, a very important structure which controls the entire hormonal system by influencing the 'master gland' itself -- the pituitary.

From this, it may be easier to understand how odours influence both the physical and emotional aspects of our being. Take the aroma of your favourite food, for example: the delicious vapour will stimulate your appetite by making your mouth water and at the same time causing the digestive juices to flow. If it is a special festive dish, all the better, for you will have many joyful memories to savour as well.

Incidentally, a healthy olfactory centre can detect over 10,000 different odours. Yet when we are subjected to the same odour for even a short while, our sense of smell becomes quickly exhausted: the olfactory cells become 'saturated' and cease to detect the odour, although we might experience a fleeting reminder of its presence from time to time. Yet it is also true that if we dislike an odour it will linger for an eternity!

Colours and Shapes

As we have already seen, aroma can evoke memories and emotions, but for some it may also suggest colours and shapes. This is a fascinating connection.

Like primary colours, all odours fall into several basic categories: floral (roses), minty (peppermint), camphoraceous or resinous (camphor), ethereal (pears), musky (musk), foul (rotten eggs) and acrid (vinegar). In the late 1940s, British chemist J.E. Amoore put forward his *stereochemical* theory of odour. Apparently, there is a connection between the geometric shape of an odoriferous molecule and the odour it produces. Using the 'lock and key' analogy, when an odoriferous molecule comes into contact with a corresponding receptor site on an olfactory neurone, it triggers a nerve impulse to the brain. For example, floral odours have a disc-shaped molecule with a tail, which fits a bowl-and-trough site. Camphoraceous odours have a spherical molecule that fits into an elliptical site, whereas minty odours have a wedge-shaped molecule that fits into a V-shaped site. Some odours fit more than one site at the same time, producing a bouquet effect.

To my nose, patchouli essence smells square with the dark hue of moist earth. Rose otto makes me think of a pinky-peach oval, whereas the odour of sweaty socks is sandy coloured with numerous floating triangles. How do you perceive odours?

The Subjectivity of Aroma

As you may have discovered, the same perfume, aftershave, cologne or whatever, smells slightly different on different people. This is because the aromatic substance interacts with our own individual body scent. No two people smell exactly alike, though there are similarities between races. Moreover, as we grow older, our bodies secrete different pheromones (subtle scent chemicals), which also appear to influence our aroma

13

preference. Consequently, a favourite perfume of our youth may seem totally obnoxious to us in maturity. As a matter of interest, during the sixteenth century valerian was a popular perfume, yet to the modern nose, it stinks! However, it would have harmonized nicely with the secretions (excretions?) of the infrequently washed bodies of the era.

Another point of interest: many normal people have 'blind spots' to certain odours or nuances of individual odours, especially to some musks. Yet others can detect odours that some people fail to perceive at all.

At Warwick University (England), Drs Steve Van Toller and George Dodd have been researching into the relationship between smell and emotion. Of the many aroma trials carried out, one is of particular note: that the skin can respond to odours — even those we cannot smell. One substance used was the sex pheromone excreted in the urine of the boar. Surprisingly, many people had a *specific anosmia* to the pheromone, i.e. they could not smell it. This included people whose sense of smell in other respects was very acute. During the experiments, volunteers were wired up to an EEG (electroencephalagram) machine which records brainwave patterns and skin responses. Very clear skin responses to the pheromone were recorded — even in those who said they could not detect the odour. Those who could smell the pheromone either loved it or hated it.

The pheromone experiment puts me in mind of the effects of sandalwood oil: people can sometimes have a specific anosmia to the entire aroma or perhaps only be able to smell an aspect of it. While some may love what they perceive as the sweet dulcet tones of the oil, others may find it repugnant, detecting a 'sweaty' note.

Incidentally, I have recently discovered a similar pheno-menon, not with an essential oil, but with the Himalayan balsam (*Impatiens glandulifera*), a plant commonly found growing wild near rivers and streams. The flowers of this plant are used in the preparation of the Bach Flower Remedy *Impatiens* (see Chapter 9). According to my nose, and to the noses of most people I know, the delicate pinkish-purple flowers are

14

odourless. However, to my discerning partner, the odour of the Himalayan balsam is truly obnoxious, causing him to respond with a gut-felt 'Ugh!' Yet surprisingly, unlike most people, he cannot always detect the sickly sweet and musky aroma of tom cat!

With the use of EEG machines, scientists have observed that certain essential oils have a specific effect on the mind or central nervous system. Some may stimulate clarity of thought (rosemary, basil, peppermint); others may have a predominantly sedative or anti-depressant effect (rose, neroli, lavender). However, the conclusion drawn from other aroma trials carried out at Warwick is that if we dislike an aroma, we are able to block its effect on the central nervous system. This supports the case for using only the essential oils we like best for aromatherapy treatments, especially for healing distressing states of mind.

Indeed, even before the scientific evidence became available, many aromatherapists knew intuitively that aroma preference is vital, for we are instinctively drawn to the fragrance of an essential oil which will be right for our needs at the time. Moreover, as our physical and emotional state alters, so might our aroma preference.

It would be no exaggeration to suggest that aromatherapy, particularly aromatherapy massage, is one of the finest treatments available for those suffering from stress or *distress*. For emotional disharmony is at root of almost all our ills. According to the visionary physician Dr Edward Bach, disease is a consolidation of a mental state. In this view he was sharing the opinion of Hippocrates as well as that of many con-temporary practitioners of holistic or whole person therapy.

Aroma, Vibration and the Mindbody

15 The human ear may be 'deaf' to high and low frequency sound, but as every physicist knows, it does not mean they do not exist, nor that we cannot be affected by them. Similarly, as discovered at Warwick, we can respond both physically and emotionally

to highly diluted fragrances, even though we may not be able to smell them. Could it be that we are responding to the subtle vibration of the aroma? If so, we might compare this to the action of homoeopathic and Bach Flower Remedies. These remedies are so highly diluted that only the energy pattern or vibration of the original medicinal material remains in the lactose tablet (homoeopathy) or the liquid (Bach Flowers). Yet if the correct remedy is chosen, the healing effect on both body and mind can be remarkable — and I can testify to this.

In fact, the French immunobiologist Dr Jacques Benveniste recently conducted convincing trials in his own laboratory which gave credence to the principle of homoeopathy. The homoeopath seeks to heal the body by administering infinitesimal quantities of a substance which, if given in material doses, causes similar symptoms to the disease which it is employed to heal. Benveniste's experiments have been replicated in laboratories all over the world. However, despite their impeccable research, he and his colleagues found themselves the target of a ferocious attack from certain members of the medical establishment who, according to Dr Julian Kenyon of The Centre for Complementary Medicine (England), were suffering from 'belief system block'. Much to their chagrin, Benveniste's findings defied the laws of materialism.

The Bach Flower Remedies take a step further into the non-material realm of 'mind over matter'. These remedies are prescribed solely for emotional disharmony (see Chapter 9).

But is there any scientific evidence to support the 'mind over matter' stance?

For centuries philosophers have contemplated the nature of mind. Some have concluded that it is a phenomenon apart from physical reality, an aspect of the immortal spirit of the individual. Others have decided that mind is merely a function of the brain; it cannot exist without the body. Although we may never know the absolute truth, modern science has begun to move closer towards understanding the essence of mind.

In the 1970s, a series of important discoveries began which centred on a new class of minute chemicals called neuro-transmitters and neuro-peptides. These chemicals were considered revolutionary at the time because they proved that the nerves did not work electrically like a telegraph system, as had been believed, but that nerve impulses were chemical in nature. Amazing as it may seem, it appears that these brain chemicals are the end products of thought. In other words, it is the *non-material* thought gives rise to the neuro-chemicals!

In the words of Dr Deepak Chopra, author of *Quantum Healing*, 'To think is to practice brain chemistry, promoting a cascade of responses throughout the body.' Moreover, receptors for neuro-chemicals are to be found in other parts of the body, for example the skin, and on cells in the immune system called monocytes. These 'intelligent' blood cells circulate freely throughout the body, apparently sending and receiving messages just as diverse as those in the central nervous system. This means that if, when we are happy, depressed, angry, in love or whatever, we produce brain chemicals in various parts of the body, then those parts also must be happy, depressed, angry or in love. Furthermore, as if this were not astonishing enough, insulin, a hormone always associated with the pancreas, is now known to be produced in the brain as well, just as brain chemicals such as transferon and CCK are produced in the stomach. Without doubt, the interrelated *mindbody* is a reality.

However, this does not explain the origin of thought which, as we have seen, appears to reside both 'outside' and 'inside' the body. Indeed, we might say thought is everywhere at once! Could it be that mind energy is an interrelated aspect of an even greater vibration, that which we might call the Universal Mind?

A well-known mathematical formula, Bell's theorem, formulated in 1964 by Irish physicist John Bell, holds that the reality of the universe is an interconnected whole wherein all objects and events respond to one another's changes in state. British astronomer Sir Arthur Eddington went so far as to conclude that an *intelligent* force holds the universe together: 'The stuff of the world is mind stuff.' More recently, British physicist David Bohm reached a similar conclusion: that there is an invisible field holding all of reality together, a field that possesses the property of knowing what is happening everywhere at once. This is the quantum mechanical world, a world beyond the proton, electron and quark — all of which can be broken down into smaller particles (at least in theory) and therefore occupy space. Whatever it is that shapes the universe and bestows it with life is *non*-material — it takes up no space. It is believed, therefore, that the quantum or subatomic world is that of energy or vibration, and it is at this point of realization that the marriage of science and mysticism takes place. Modern physics, in tune with Eastern mysticism, pictures the universe as a continuous, dancing and vibrating web of life.

In the quantum realm, there is no distinction between animate and inanimate, between spirit and matter. We might say we perceive them as separate because they vibrate at different frequencies. Mind energy, for instance, vibrates so fast that it appears to be invisible, whereas rock vibrates so slowly that we are unaware of its essential dynamism.

Where does aroma fit into this picture, in particular, the essential oils of plants? They could be seen as a rainbow bridge linking the 'two worlds' of spirit and matter. With essential oils we have not only the material substance of the oil, with its therapeutic properties, which vibrates at a similar frequency to that of the body, but we also have the ethereal aroma, which influences us on a much more subtle level. As the great philosopher Rudolph Steiner said, 'Matter is the most spiritual in the perfume of the plant.' Could a pleasing fragrance be vibrating in harmony with the spiritual aspect of our being? After all, it is a law of physics that like attracts like, a principle which is also known in science as *resonance*.

Aromatic Signatures

Let us conclude this chapter with one final thought on the subject of aroma and vibration. It may come as a surprise to learn that no two people can create an identical-smelling aromatherapy oil, even when they use the same combination of oils in the exact quantities and from the same bottles. The oils always take on an aspect of our character or mood; they literally become imbibed with our 'personal vibes'. Carry out the little experiment suggested on pages 90–1, and see for yourself!

2 · The Essence of the Art

Essential oils are the odoriferous liquid components of aromatic plants, trees and grasses. They are sometimes called 'ethereal oils', a Germanic term which aptly describes their Otherworldly nature; for if left in the open air they disappear without a trace, evaporating into the ether like a faerie mist.

The oils are contained in tiny oil glands or sacs which are concentrated in different parts of the plant. They may be found in the petals (rose), the leaves (eucalyptus), the roots of grass (vetiver), the heart wood (sandalwood), the fruit (lemon), the seeds (caraway), the rhizomes (ginger), the resin (pine) and sometimes in more than one part of the plant. Lavender, for instance, yields an oil from both flowers and leaves. The orange tree is particularly interesting for it produces three different-smelling essences with differing therapeutic properties: the heady bitter-sweet neroli (flowers), the similar, though less refined, scent of petitgrain (leaves) and the cheery orange (skin of the fruit).

The more oil glands or sacs present in the plant, the cheaper the oil and vice versa. For instance, 100 kilos of lavender yields almost 3 litres of essential oil, whereas 100 kilos of rose petals can yield only half a litre of oil. Although some essences are very expensive, especially rose otto and neroli, they are highly concentrated substances; if used correctly, as advocated in this book, you will find that a little goes a long way.

Plant essences may be technically classified as oils, but they are in fact quite different from ordinary 'fixed oils' such as corn or sunflower. Because they are highly volatile they do not leave a permanent mark on paper, and unlike fatty vegetable oils, most essences have the consistency of water or alcohol and are not at all greasy. They are soluble in wax (melted beeswax or jojoba for example), egg yolk, alcohol and vegetable oils. Even though they are not entirely soluble in water, they can be used most successfully in the bath if the water is agitated to disperse the fine droplets.

Extracting Essential Oils

The most classic method of extraction is steam distillation, which is a sophisticated version of an ancient method first devised in Mesopotamia over 5,000 years ago. Plant material is piled into a still and subjected to concentrated steam, which acts to release the essential oils from the plant cells. The aromatic vapour travels along a series of glass tubes which form a condenser. The oil is then easily separated from the water by being siphoned off through a narrow-necked container. The remaining water may form a beautifully fragrant by-product: rosewater, orange flower water and lavender water are well-known examples.

A more recent innovation is vacuum distillation. By reducing air pressure in the sealed distillation apparatus, a vacuum is created. Distillation is thus achieved at much lower temperatures, which preserves the delicate flower fragrances more successfully.

The essences of citrus fruits such as orange, lemon, bergamot and mandarin are found in the rind, so these can be obtained by a simple process known as *expression*. Although this was once carried out by hand (by squeezing the rind), machines using centrifugal force are now used instead.

A virtually obsolete method of extraction is called *enfleurage*. Here, animal fat, usually lard, is used to absorb the essences, which are then separated from the fat by alcohol. Essences readily dissolve in alcohol, but fat does not. The alcohol is then evaporated off, leaving behind the essential oil. This method is still employed by some perfumiers to capture the fragrances of flowers such as jasmine, orange flower and tuberose whose exquisite fragrances would be spoiled by the intense heat of distillation. If you can actually find such an extraction, it will be labelled '*enfleurage* absolute', not 'essential oil', and will cost a fortune! Very few (if any) of these *enfleurage* absolutes reach the essential oil suppliers. Of course, the use of animal fat will be off-putting to many. Beeswax or vegetable oil could be used instead, but I have yet to come across such a product.

The high cost of this labour-intensive and time-consuming method has led to the wide use of solvents such as hexane and petroleum ether as a means of capturing the essences of the aforementioned flowers. These oils, which are widely available from essential oil suppliers, are labelled 'absolute' and, though more expensive than most essential oils (with the exception of rose otto), they are not as costly as the *enfleurage* absolutes mentioned earlier.

The most recent method is low-temperature carbon-dioxide extraction, which results in some exquisite aromas. Though an expensive process, it is of great interest to those who would prefer to avoid solvent extracted absolutes. Quite apart from concern over traces of solvent often left behind in absolutes, we cannot ignore the environmental effects of these substances being discharged into the atmosphere as well as possibly being absorbed by distillery workers. Carbon-dioxide extraction is generally regarded as a cleaner alternative to the use of potentially toxic solvents.

Organically Produced Oils

Unfortunately, very few essential oils are produced by organic methods, that is to say, extracted from plants grown without the use of chemical fertilizers and poisonous sprays. The oils that are labelled 'organic' tend to be of the herb variety — oils such as lavender, rosemary, marjoram and camomile — though some oils, particularly those from trees such as sandalwood, frankincense and myrrh, are imported from countries where chemical sprays and fertilizers are not in general use. However, if you care about the environment, it is best to avoid rosewood essence (sometimes called *bois de rose*). Unfortunately, this oil is extracted from trees that are torn down from the rapidly diminishing rainforests of South America and also Africa.

The Properties of Essential Oils

An aromatic plant produces essential oils for its own survival: to influence growth and reproduction, to attract pollinating insects, to repel predators and to protect itself from disease — and they can do as much for people too.

Studies have shown that essential oils of lavender and neroli, for example, promote the growth of healthy skin cells. Others, such as fennel, rose and cypress, influence hormonal secretions, thus exerting a beneficial effect on the human reproductive system. Many oils, notably rosemary, geranium and eucalyptus, will kill head lice (the equivalent to an attack of greenfly!), and oils such as tea tree, garlic and thyme actually strengthen the immune system. Indeed, I know of a case in Australia whereby a man recovered from full-blown AIDS as a result of naturopathic treatment which included the use of these oils.[1] As for 'attracting pollinating insects', for centuries essential oils such as sandalwood, rose otto, ylang ylang and patchouli have been credited with aphrodisiac properties! Although it is possible that they may have a direct hormonal influence, it is more likely that they work on a subtle level, influencing the mind and emotions through the sense of smell.

However, when using essential oils to help emotional states, do remember that it is important to love the fragrance; the mind is far more powerful than the aroma of an essential oil. If you dislike the aroma, the treatment will be completely ruined.

All essential oils are antiseptic; some are endowed with anti-viral properties as well, notably eucalyptus, garlic and tea tree. Unlike harsh chemical antiseptics, essential oils, if used correctly, are harmless to tissue, yet they are powerful aggressors towards germs. Dr Jean Valnet (one of the French pioneers of aromatherapy) used essential oils to treat the horrific wounds of soldiers during the Second World War. Not only did the fragrances of the essences cover up the putrid smell of gangrenous wounds, but they also retarded putrefaction. Moreover, Valnet observed that the troops who slept rough

1. See *International Journal of Aromatherapy* (1988), Vol. 1, No.3.

in pine forests suffered from fewer respiratory complaints as a result of the pine resin whose vapour saturated the air. Similarly, Swiss sanatoriums are traditionally sited near pine forests to help those suffering from bronchial complaints and tuberculosis.

Interestingly, Jean Valnet and other pioneers discovered that blends of certain essential oils are not only more powerful than when the oils are used singly, but that the mysterious factor of synergy is at work — the whole becoming greater than the sum of its equal parts. This is particularly noticeable with the anti-bacterial action of essences. A blend of clove, thyme, lavender and peppermint, for example, is far more powerful than a chemist might expect of the blend (taking into account the combined chemical constituents of the oils). Curiously, however, mixing more than five essences is counter-productive, rather like a discordant musical chord. The anti-bacterial action is then weakened.

Essential oils also act on the central nervous system — some will relax (camomile, neroli), others will stimulate (rosemary, black pepper). A few have the ability to 'normalize'. Garlic, for instance, can raise low blood pressure and lower high blood pressure when taken internally in the form of garlic capsules. Likewise, bergamot and geranium can either sedate or stimulate, according to individual needs — a phenomenon totally alien to a synthetic drug.

Studies have also shown that essential oils have a very small molecular structure, which enables them to pass through the skin's hair follicles, which contain sebum, an oily liquid with which they have an affinity. From here they diffuse into the bloodstream or are taken up by the lymph and interstitial fluid (a liquid surrounding all body cells) to other parts of the body. If the skin is healthy, it takes about an hour for the oil to be absorbed; much longer if the skin is congested or if there is much subcutaneous fat. At the same time, when inhaled, the aromatic molecules reach the lungs, from where they diffuse across the tiny air sacs into the surrounding blood capillaries and then into the general bloodstream.

Whether absorbed through the skin or inhaled, once in the

bloodstream and body fluids, the essences exert their therapeutic effect — even though the amount absorbed is very small indeed. However, the efficacy of the oils may be due to the fact that aromatherapy treatments are given once or twice weekly over a period of not less than one month. This acts to gently stimulate the mindbody's innate self-healing ability. We also know that essential oils, having triggered their healing effect, are rapidly excreted from the body. Therefore, if used correctly, there is little danger of toxicity. However, essential oils should never be taken by mouth, except under the strict guidance of a qualified clinical aromatherapist or other suitably qualified practitioner.

The chemistry of essential oils is complex. They may consist of hundreds of constituents such as terpenes, alcohols, aldehydes, esters and, no doubt, many other as yet undiscovered constituents. This explains why a single essential oil can help a wide variety of disorders. A synthetic drug, on the other hand, may contain a single, therefore an unbalanced, but very powerful, active principle. Moreover, synthetic drugs lack the synergistic action of an essential oil or herbal medicine. As a result, they tend to act in the manner of the proverbial 'sledge-hammer to crack a nut'. Adverse side-effects are the inevitable outcome of such an onslaught. Essential oils, on the other hand, work *with* the body, strengthening its own natural defences — especially when used in conjunction with a healthy diet and sensible lifestyle.

However, we need to adopt a balanced viewpoint and accept that the use of drugs cannot be totally ruled out; everything has its place. If, for example, a person fails to respond to natural treatment and is in a great deal of discomfort, or in life or death situations (road accidents, congenital organ dysfunction and so forth) drug intervention may be vital.

Although chemists have tried to duplicate essential oils in the laboratory, the results are not the same. A synthetic chemical is, in theory, identical to that found in nature; in practice, as every chemist knows, it is impossible to make a 100 per cent pure chemical. Any synthetic chemical will carry with it a small percentage of undesirable substances which are not found in the essential oil. Although many synthetic aromatic oils have certain therapeutic properties in common with the natural substance, from my own experience, these oils are far more likely to cause allergies. Above all, however, no synthetic compound can reproduce the naturally occurring vibration or energy pattern of the 'stuff of life'.

Buying Essential Oils

It is essential that only pure, unadulterated essential oils are used in therapy. Most aromatherapists obtain their oils from reputable mail order suppliers (see pages 158–60), not from shops concerned with beauty and perfumery. The advantages offered by mail order suppliers over retail outlets includes a wider range of oils and lower prices on larger quantities. Though if you are new to aromatherapy, it may be best to buy your oils from a health shop or from a well respected herbal supplier. This will give you the opportunity of smelling the oils first, and buying only those you like.

Most important:
Do check that an essential oil labelled as such is in fact 100 per cent essential oil and not one that has been diluted in almond oil (this is sometimes the case with expensive oils such as rose or neroli).

Caring for your Oils

Storage is important. Essential oils should be sold in well-stoppered dark glass bottles and stored away from light, heat and damp. Avoid essential oils sold in bottles with a rubber-tipped dropper. Certain essential oils, cedarwood in particular, can cause rubber to perish into a sticky mess. Despite this rather alarming fact, essential oils are harmless to skin if used correctly as outlined in this book.

In theory, most essential oils will keep for several years — except for the citrus oils, which begin to deteriorate after about six months. Bergamot essence, however, will keep for up to two

25

years. A few oils will improve with age, rather like some good wines; examples of these are sandalwood, frankincense, rose otto and patchouli. In fact, a 20-year-old patchouli essence will be extremely mellow and fragrant, and there is even a market for vintage frankincense! However, the more often you open the bottle of any essential oil, the greater the chance of oxidation and thus of reduction in the oil's therapeutic properties. If stored carefully though, in a cool, dark place (preferably in an old fridge kept for this purpose, especially if you have a large selection of oils), they will keep for *at least* one year — from one harvest to the next — with no problem at all. Once diluted in vegetable oil, however (for use as a massage oil), essential oils will keep for no longer than two months, perhaps three if kept in a cool place.

Using Essential Oils

The main methods for using essential oils are to be found in subsequent chapters. Suffice it to say here, they can be used in a variety of ways to promote health and vitality. They can be blended with the finest vegetable oils, waxes and floral waters to be used as superb skin care agents. They can be added to the bath, used in steam inhalations for colds and 'flu, or blended into intriguing mood-enhancing perfumes and massage oils. They can also be vaporized to create an enjoyable ambience in the home — and much more besides. Before we look at the techniques of aromatherapy, in the following chapter we shall take a closer look at the therapeutic properties of a number of the most commonly used essential oils.

3 · Essential Oil Profiles

The essential oils described here are some of those most commonly used in aromatherapy. The main therapeutic properties of the oils are listed. However, when choosing oils to help emotional disharmony, do be guided by your aroma preference. Aromatherapy is meant to be enjoyable. In fact, the more wonderful the experience, the more healing its effect. Aroma preference is less important when using oils for the symptomatic treatment of problems such as athlete's foot or sprains — though some aromatherapists would disagree. Each essential oil has a myriad of therapeutic properties, so it should not be too difficult to find an oil (or a blend of oils) to suit your aroma preference as well as your physical ailment. If, however, you are suffering from a long-term problem such as arthritis, asthma, eczema or chronic nervous tension, do seek expert advice from a qualified health practitioner, aromatherapist or counsellor, preferably someone with a knowledge of holistic healing principles. Diet and lifestyle play an important role in our physical and emotional well-being.

Of course, you need not be ill to enjoy aromatherapy — the oils can be used purely for pleasure. However, before using any essential oil, please check that it is safe for you to use. Some oils should not be used during pregnancy, for instance. Where appropriate, a 'Caution' note is included at the end of an essential oil profile.

Important:
It is advisable to use oils in half the stated quantities during pregnancy and also for children under 12. Never use essential oils for babies or young children except under the strict guidance of a qualified aromatherapist. Essential oils are very powerful, so need to be used with care. Never use an essential oil about which you can find little or no information.

A Word about Allergies

It is possible to be allergic to almost anything — even to the seemingly innocuous sweet almond oil. A few people may be skin-sensitive to oils such as peppermint, basil, bergamot, ylang ylang, lemongrass, camomile, melissa, geranium or ginger, especially if used in a high concentration.

If you suffer from asthma, never use steam inhalations (with or without essential oils). Concentrated steam may trigger an attack.

If you are one of the rare people allergic to all essential oils, unfortunately you will have to try another therapy such as herbal medicine or homoeopathy.

Recommended concentrations of the oils are given in Chapter 6.

The Essential Oils

BASIL
Ocimum basilicum

Source:	Distillation of the leaves and flowering tops from the herb native to southern Asia and the Middle East.
Aroma:	Agreeably spicy, vaguely reminiscent of cloves.
Blends well with:	Bergamot and other citrus oils, frankincense, geranium, neroli.
Uses:	Primarily a nerve tonic and a mental stimulant. Helps bronchitis, colds, coughs, headache, mental and physical fatigue, scanty menstrual periods, sinus problems.
CAUTION:	Not to be used during pregnancy. To be avoided if you have sensitive skin. Always use in the lowest concentrations.

28

BERGAMOT
Citrus bergamia

Source:	Obtained by expression of the rind of the small orange-like fruit native to Italy.
Aroma:	Delightfully citrus with a slightly spicy overtone.
Blends well with:	Most other essences, particularly geranium, lavender, ylang ylang.
Uses:	Primarily uplifting and anti-depressant. A 'balancing' oil capable of relaxing or stimulating according to individual needs. Helpful for boils, cold sores, cystitis, fevers, oily skin conditions, pre-menstrual syndrome, tonsilitis (as a gargle: put 4 drops in a teacupful of warm water and use two or three times a day).
CAUTION:	Not to be used on the skin immediately before sunbathing, as it may cause permanent pigmentation. However, it is now possible to obtain bergaptene-free bergamot essence, labelled 'Bergamot FCF', which will not react on the skin in sunlight. As a skin oil, it is advisable to use this essence in a moderate to low concentration.

BLACK PEPPER
Piper nigrum

Source:	Distillation of the fruit (berries). A woody climber native to Malaysia and South East Asia.
Aroma:	Hot and spicy, just like freshly milled black pepper.
Blends well with:	Citrus essences, frankincense, patchouli, sandalwood, vetiver.
Uses:	Primarily a stimulating essence, both physically and mentally. Helpful for cellulite,

Uses (continued): colic, constipation, coughs, 'flu, muscular aches and pains, poor circulation, stomach pains.

CAUTION: Not to be used as a facial oil as it may be too strong.

CAMOMILE, ROMAN
Anthemis noblis

Source: Distillation of the dried daisy-like flowers. The herb is native to northern Europe.

Aroma: Unusual, dry and slightly sweet — often described as smelling like apples, but not to my nose!

Blends well with: Citrus essences, geranium, lavender, rose, ylang ylang.

Uses: Primarily anti–inflammatory (due to a high content of azulene) and sedative. Helpful for acne, allergies (skin and respiratory), anxiety, boils, chilblains, cold sores, colic, colitis, eczema, indigestion, insomnia, menopausal problems, migraine, neuralgia, period pain, pre-menstrual syndrome, psoriasis, rheumatism, skin care (most skins), sprains, stomach cramps, thread veins, wounds, inflammation of joints, swellings.

CAUTION: A very powerful essence which is best used in the lowest concentrations, especially when treating allergies.

CEDARWOOD
Juniperus virginiana

Source: Distillation of the wood shavings from the evergreen tree native to North America.

Aroma: Woody, reminiscent of pencils!

Blends well with: Bergamot, clary sage, cypress, juniper, neroli, rose.

Uses:	Acts primarily on the skin and the respiratory tract; has diuretic properties. Helpful for acne, anxiety, bronchitis, catarrh, coughs, cystitis, dandruff, eczema (use in ½ per cent concentrations), oily skin conditions, premenstrual syndrome, as an insect repellent.
CAUTION:	Not to be used during pregnancy.

CINNAMON BARK
Cinnamomum zeylancium

Source:	Distillation of the bark chips from the small tree native to Sri Lanka, India and Madagascar.
Aroma:	Warm and spicy, similar to good quality powdered cinnamon. You may also find cinnamon *leaf*, which has a less refined aroma.
Blends well with:	Cedarwood, citrus essences, cloves, coriander, ginger, rose otto, sandalwood.
Uses:	A warming, anti-depressant, antibiotic, anti-viral oil. Use as room fragrance, or as a fumigant during infectious illness.
CAUTION:	This oil is a powerful skin irritant. *Use only as a vaporizing essence.*

CLARY SAGE
Salvia sclarea

Source:	Distillation of the flowering leaves and tops from the herb native to the Mediterranean.
Aroma:	Sweet and warmly floral, very different from the herby aroma of common sage (*Salvia officinalis*).
Blends well with:	Cedarwood, citrus essences, cypress, frankincense, geranium, lavender, marjoram, neroli, petitgrain, sandalwood, vetiver.
Uses:	Primarily a nerve tonic, warming and sedative. Helpful for absence of periods

outside pregnancy, anxiety, boils, excessive perspiration, high blood pressure, insect bites and stings, insomnia, leucorrhoea, nervous tension, painful periods, pre-menstrual syndrome, throat infections, whooping cough.

CAUTION: Not to be used during pregnancy.

CLOVE
Eugenia caryophyllata

Source: Distillation of the flower buds of the small evergreen tree which is native to Madagascar.

Aroma: Very strong and bittersweet, unmistakable.

Blends well with: Cinnamon bark, citrus oils, especially orange.

Uses: As a room fragrance/fumigant or as an analgesic for toothache. (Put one drop of the neat essence into the tooth cavity, or put a few drops on a damp cotton bud and apply to the gums, around the aching tooth.)

CAUTION: This oil is a powerful skin irritant, so use only as a vaporizing essence or as a first-aid measure for toothache. Never use neat as a long-term remedy as the essence may damage the gums. Seek dental treatment as soon as possible. Avoid during pregnancy.

CORIANDER
Coriandrum sativum

Source: Distillation of the fruit (the so-called seeds). A herb indigenous to southern Europe.

Aroma: Agreeably piquant and fruity.

Blends well with: Citrus oils, cypress, juniper, marjoram, petitgrain.

Uses: Generally warming and stimulating to the mind. Formerly held to be an aphrodisiac. Helpful for colic, depression, loss of appetite, mental fatigue, nervous debility, rheumatism.

CYPRESS
Cupressus sempervirens

Source:	Distillation of the leaves and fruit (cones). A tall conical-shaped tree native to the East and the Mediterranean.
Aroma:	A cooling, somewhat solemn aroma, similar to pine.
Blends well with:	Cedarwood, citrus oils, clary sage, lavender, marjoram, petitgrain, pine needle, sandalwood.
Uses:	Primarily astringent, mentally clearing and mildly sedative. Helpful for anxiety and nervous tension, bronchitis, cellulite, diarrhoea, excessive perspiration, 'flu, haemorrhoids, heavy periods, incontinence, loss of voice, menopausal problems, oily skin conditions, painful periods, pyorrhoea of the gums, rheumatism, spasmodic coughs, thread veins, varicose veins.

EUCALYPTUS
Eucalyptus globulus

Source:	Distillation of the leaves of a tall tree native to Australia.
Aroma:	Camphoraceous.
Blends well with:	Lavender, lemon, pine, sandalwood.
Uses:	A powerful antiseptic with a marked effect on the respiratory system. Helpful for allergies to animal fur, bronchitis, burns, catarrh, cold sores, colds, coughs, cystitis, diabetes (can lower excess blood sugar levels), fevers, 'flu, hayfever, head lice, leucorrhoea, measles, migraine, neuralgia, rheumatism, scarlet fever, sinusitis, sprains, throat infections, ulcers of the skin, wounds, as an insect repellent.

FRANKINCENSE
Boswellia thurifera

Source:	Distillation of the hardened resin ('tears') of the small north African tree.
Aroma:	Warm and balsamic.
Blends well with:	Basil, black pepper, cedarwood, citrus essences, coriander, lavender, myrrh, neroli, rose, sandalwood, vetiver.
Uses:	Highly valued for its effects on the mind, especially when used as a meditation aid, and for its effect on the respiratory tract. Helpful for acne, bronchitis, catarrh, coughs, deep wounds, haemorrhoids, lethargy, nose bleeds, skin care (particularly ageing skin).

GERANIUM
Pelargonium odorantissium

Source:	Distillation of the whole plant native to Reunion, Madagascar and Guinea.
Aroma:	Freshly floral and sweet.
Blends well with:	Most other essences, especially bergamot, neroli, petitgrain, ylang ylang.
Uses:	Like bergamot, geranium is a balancing essence, capable of relaxing or stimulating according to individual needs. Helpful for cellulite, diabetes (like eucalyptus, it can lower excessive blood sugar levels), fluid retention, mouth ulcers, neuralgia, ringworm, shingles, sore throats, thrush, wounds.
CAUTION:	Although a balancing oil for most people, I have known this oil to be too stimulating for a few sensitive individuals. Moreover, some breastfeeding mothers who have used the oil on their skin have reported that it sometimes has a stimulating effect on babies.

34

GINGER
Zingiber officinale

Source:	Distillation of the roots (rhizomes) of the plant native to China.
Aroma:	Not as pleasantly pungent as the freshly grated root. Unfortunately, the intense heat of distillation tends to distort the aroma.
Blends well with:	Citrus oils, coriander, patchouli, vetiver. But go easy, otherwise its powerful aroma will dominate your blends.
Uses:	Warming to both body and mind. A reputed aphrodisiac. Helpful for arthritis, chilblains, colds, cramp, fibrositis, 'flu, muscle sprain, muscular aches and pains, nervous tension and anxiety, poor circulation, rheumatism, travel sickness, as a gargle for sore throats (1 or 2 drops in a cup of water, stir well).
CAUTION:	Not suitable for those with sensitive skin. Avoid during pregnancy as it may be too stimulating.

JUNIPER
Juniperus communis

Source:	Distillation of the berries from the evergreen shrub native to the northern hemisphere. There is also an inferior grade oil obtained from the wood.
Aroma:	Clear, slightly peppery, with a resinous overtone.
Blends well with:	Citrus essences, geranium, lavender, rosemary, sandalwood.
Uses:	Primarily tonic, cleansing and diuretic. Helpful for absence of periods outside pregnancy, arthritis, cellulite, coughs, cystitis, fluid retention, gout, haemorrhoids, nervous tension, oily skin conditions, respiratory infections, rheumatism, weeping eczema.

CAUTION: It is important to differentiate between 'Juniper Berry' and 'Juniper' — the latter is usually the inferior grade. The oil should be labelled 'J. Berry'. Medicinal properties are reduced in the oil obtained from the wood. Not to be used during pregnancy.

LAVENDER
Lavandula officinalis

Source: Distillation of the leaves and flowering tops. The plant is native to the Mediterranean.

Aroma: Refreshingly floral.

Blends well with: Most essences, especially bergamot, camomile, clary sage, frankincense, juniper, marjoram, rose, ylang ylang.

Uses: Regulates the central nervous system. Helpful for abscess, acne, athlete's foot, anxiety, boils, bronchitis, burns, chilblains, colds, coughs, cuts, cystitis, dandruff, depression, earache, eczema, fainting, flatulence, fluctuating moods, head lice, high blood pressure, infectious illness, insect bites and stings, insomnia, laryngitis, leucorrhoea, migraine, muscular aches and pains, nervous tension, periods (scanty and painful), pre-menstrual syndrome, skin care (all skin types), sprains, as a hair tonic.

LEMON
Citrus limonum

Source: Expression of the lemon rind. The lemon tree is native to the Mediterranean.

Aroma: Clear, sharp and refreshing. The essential oil does not keep well; use within six to nine months.

Blends well with: Most essences, especially camomile,

eucalyptus, fennel, frankincense, geranium, juniper, lavender, pine, tea tree, ylang ylang.

Uses: Fortifying to the nervous system. Helpful for anaemia, arthritis, cellulite, chilblains, colds, 'flu, fluid retention, gallstones, high blood pressure, insect bites and stings, rheumatism, sore throats, verrucae, warts, wounds, as an insect repellent.

CAUTION: Not to be used on the skin prior to sunbathing. It may cause permanent pigmentation.

MARJORAM, SWEET
Origanum marjorana

Source: Distillation of the flowering tops and leaves from the herb native to Hungary.

Aroma: Warm and vaguely spicy.

Blends well with: Bergamot, coriander, lavender.

Uses: Warming and calming to the nervous system. Helpful for anxiety, arthritis, bronchitis, bruises, colds, constipation, flatulence, headaches, high blood pressure, indigestion, leucorrhoea, migraine, muscular aches and pains, nervous tension, painful periods.

CAUTION: Not to be used during pregnancy.

MYRRH
Commiphora myrrha

Source: Distillation of the gum which is exuded from the small tree native to north-east Africa.

Aroma: A warm, dry balsamic aroma — rather medicinal.

3 7

Blends well with: Cedarwood, citrus essences, cypress, frankincense, juniper, neroli, patchouli, petitgrain, rose, sandalwood, vetiver.

Uses: Primarily antiseptic and anti-inflammatory.

	Helpful for absence of periods outside pregnancy, bronchitis, catarrh, coughs, diarrhoea, flatulence, gingivitis, haemorrhoids, mouth ulcers, pyrrhoea of the gums, skin care (particularly ageing sin), skin ulcers, thrush, wounds.
Note:	Myrrh tends to harden, so you may have to leave the bottle in a cup of hot water for a few minutes until it has softened enough for easy use.
CAUTION:	Not to be used during pregnancy.

NEROLI
Citrus aurantium, bigaradia

Source:	Distillation of the blossom from the bitter orange tree native to southern Europe.
Aroma:	A sweetish dry scent, not at all 'citrusy'.
Blends well with:	Camomile, cedarwood, citrus essences, clary sage, cypress, frankincense, gcranium, juniper, lavender, rose, sandalwood, vetiver.
Uses:	Primarily anti-depressant and sedative with a slightly hypnotic effect. A reputed aphrodisiac. Helpful for depression, emotional shock, hysteria, insomnia, nervous tension, palpitations, skin care (suits most skins).

ORANGE
Citrus aurantium

(Oil of Mandarin, *Citrus nobilis*, has similar properties, but a sweeter, more delicate aroma.)

Source:	Expression of the rind from the fruit native to southern Europe.
Aroma:	Similar to fresh oranges, sweet and cheery. The essential oil does not keep well; use within six to nine months.

Blends well with: Coriander (and all other spices), cypress, frankincense, juniper, vetiver.

Uses: A general tonic with an uplifting aroma. Helpful for anxiety and depression, bronchitis, chills, colds.

CAUTION: Not to be applied to the skin prior to sunbathing. It may cause permanent pigmentation.

PATCHOULI
Pogostemon patchouli

Source: Distillation of the dried leaves. The herb is native to the Far East and the West Indies.

Aroma: An earthy Eastern scent which becomes sweeter once the sour element of the oil has worn off.

Blends well with: Cedarwood, citrus essences, geranium, ginger, lavender, myrrh, neroli, pine needle, rose.

Uses: Primarily antibiotic, anti-fungal, anti-depressant and fortifying. A reputed aphrodisiac. Helpful for acne, anxiety and depression, athlete's foot, cellulite, cracked skin, dandruff, fevers, fluid retention, sores, thinning hair.

PEPPERMINT
Mentha piperita

Source: Distillation of the leaves and flowering tops. The herb is native to Europe.

Aroma: Pungent and fresh.

Blends well with: Does not blend very well with other essences, unless used in small quantities, as it tends to overpower blends, but is acceptable with basil, clary sage, coriander, eucalyptus, lavender, marjoram, rosemary and tea tree.

Uses: Primarily a mental stimulant. Also helpful for

athlete's foot, bronchitis, colds, dry coughs, fainting, fevers, 'flu, headache, indigestion, migraine, nausea, scabies, sinusitis, as an insect repellent.

CAUTION: May irritate the skin if used in concentrations above 1 per cent. Best avoided during the first trimester of pregnancy as it may be too stimulating.

PETITGRAIN
Citrus aurantium

Source: Distillation of the leaves and twigs of the bitter orange tree native to southern Europe.

Aroma: Similar to neroli, but less refined and woody.

Blends well with: Bergamot and other citrus essences, clary sage, cypress, geranium, juniper, lavender, pine, rosemary, vetiver, ylang ylang.

Uses: Primarily fortifying to the nervous system. Helpful for anxiety and nervous tension, insomnia, palpitations.

PINE NEEDLE
Pinus sylvestris

Source: Distillation of pine needles. The tree is native to northern Europe. Lower grades are obtained by distillation of the cones, young twigs and branches.

Aroma: Cooling and woody.

Blends well with: Bergamot, cedarwood, lemon, patchouli, petitgrain, rosemary, sandalwood, tea tree.

Uses: Primarily antiseptic, antibiotic, diuretic and stimulating. Helpful for arthritis, bronchitis, catarrh, colds, cystitis, 'flu, laryngitis, lethargy, rheumatism, wounds. (Medicinal properties of all grades are virtually the same.)

ROSE OTTO
Rosa damascena

Source: Distillation of the flower petals. Native to Bulgaria.

Aroma: Smooth and warm with a hint of vanilla and cloves. Not to be confused with rose absolute (extracted by solvents), which is yellowy-orange and has a lighter aroma. Rose otto is virtually colourless and is semi-solid at room temperature.

Blends well with: Many essences, especially bergamot, camomile, cedarwood, clary sage, frankincense, lavender, patchouli, sandalwood, vetiver, ylang ylang. A tiny amount is all you will need as it is so concentrated.

Uses: Primarily an oil for healing distressing states of mind such as anxiety and depression. The essence is a reputed aphrodisiac. Also helpful for hangover (it has a cleansing effect on the liver), heavy or irregular periods, leucorrhoea, menopausal symptoms, pre-menstrual syndrome, respiratory disorders, skin care (especially dry, ageing), thread veins, uterine disorders.

ROSEMARY
Rosemarinus officinalis

Source: Distillation of the flowering tops of the herb native to Spain.

Aroma: Warm, sharp and camphoraceous.

Blends well with: Basil, cedarwood, citrus oils, coriander, frankincense, juniper, lavender, peppermint.

41 *Uses:* Primarily a stimulating essence to both body and mind. Helpful for arthritis, bronchitis, burns, colds, dandruff, falling hair, 'flu, headache, head lice, high cholesterol,

indigestion, low blood pressure, mental fatigue, migraine, nervous debility, palpitations, rheumatism, skin care (especially oily skin conditions), wounds.

CAUTION: Not to be used during the first trimester of pregnancy as it may be too stimulating. In very high concentrations, and if used continuously over a long period of time, it may provoke convulsions in prone subjects.

SANDALWOOD
Santalum album

Source: Distillation of the heartwood. Sandalwood is a small parasitic tree (it buries its roots in those of neighbouring trees) native to India.

Aroma: Softly woody and sweet, very tenacious.

Blends well with: Many essences, especially black pepper, frankincense, myrrh, neroli, rose, ylang ylang.

Uses: Primarily for nervous tension, respiratory disorders and skin problems. A reputed aphrodisiac. Also helpful for acne, bronchitis, catarrh, coughs, cystitis, depression, diarrhoea, insomnia, laryngitis, pre-menstrual syndrome, skin care (oily, dry or ageing skins).

TEA TREE
Melaleuca alternifolia

Source: Distillation of the leaves and twigs. A hardy tree native to Australia.

Aroma: Medicinal, reminiscent of a mixture of juniper and cypress, but less refined than these two oils.

Blends well with: Does not blend very well with other essences, but the aroma can be improved by mixing with a little eucalyptus, lemon, lavender or pine.

42

Uses: Primarily an antiseptic, antibiotic, anti-viral, anti-fungal essence. A powerful immune system stimulant. Helpful for acne, athlete's foot, cold sores, colds, coughs, dandruff, 'flu, insect bites and stings, ringworm, thrush, verrucae, warts, wounds. A few drops in the bath can soothe the effects of shock and hysteria.

VETIVER
Vetiveria zizanoides

Source: Distillation of the roots. Vetiver is a wild grass native to India.

Aroma: Rich, warm and earthy with a sweet background.

Blends well with: Citrus essences, clary sage, frankincense, geranium, ginger, myrrh, rose, ylang ylang.

Uses: Primarily an oil for healing distressing emotions. A reputed aphrodisiac. Helpful for aching muscles, extreme nervousness and stress, high blood pressure, insomnia, light-headedness (following 'flu for instance), pre-menstrual syndrome, skin care (especially ageing skin).

YLANG YLANG
Cananga odorata (pronounced *ee-lang-ee-lang*)

Source: Distillation of the flower petals of the flowering tree native to Indonesia.

Aroma: Very sweet, reminiscent of almonds and night-scented stock (*Matthiola bicornis*).

Blends well with: Camomile, cedarwood, citrus oils, geranium, lavender, patchouli, rose, sandalwood, vetiver.

Uses: Primarily an oil for healing distressing emotions. A reputed aphrodisiac. Helpful for anxiety, depression, high blood pressure, nervous tension, palpitations, pre-menstrual syndrome.

CAUTION: Try to obtain the finest quality oil, which will be listed as ylang ylang extra. Inferior grades known as ylang ylang 2, 3 or Cananga are also available. Ylang ylang extra is obtained from the 'first running' of the distillation process which continues for the subsequent grades. Once you have smelled the clarity of ylang ylang extra and compared it to inferior grades, your nose will be your guide thereafter.

4 · Aromatherapy Techniques

There are a number of enjoyable ways of using essential oils to alleviate specific health problems and to engender a sense of well-being. Aromatherapy is also a wonderful preventative treatment, for the oils act to strengthen the immune system, which can become weakened by the stresses and strains of life. Although we shall look at each aromatherapeutic technique in turn, aromatherapy massage takes pride of place, being one of the finest treatments available to soothe those suffering from stress in its many guises. However, before we go any further we need to determine what we actually mean by stress.

The Nature of Stress

Most people think of stress as being the outside pressures and problems that impinge upon us — problems such as deadlines, noise, marital strife, excessive demands made on our time by others and so forth. In actual fact, stress is our own personal reaction to those things (or people) 'out there'. We all know people who remain cool, calm and collected under the most trying circumstances, and others who collapse under the strain of even relatively minor difficulties.

However, it is also true that we need a certain amount of stimulation to motivate us and keep us going. Indeed, without the 'spice of life' we begin to feel despondent, or apathetic — life then appears bleak and meaningless. So stress only becomes a problem if it develops into *distress*. Indeed, almost all of us can recall a time in our lives when we have been distressed and have become ill as a result. Perhaps it was just a cold or possibly something more serious. Many people also become more accident prone at such times.

Whether you are suffering from the kind of stress associated with overload or from that born of a monotonous existence, regular, though moderate exercise will help enormously. Fairly strenuous activity stimulates the circulation and deepens the breathing, which in turn increases oxygen levels in the blood. This has a definite positive effect on our state of mind. Anyone who has recently taken up some form of exercise, especially something they actively enjoy, will tell you that it has brought them enhanced mental energy and concentration, the ability to sleep more deeply, and a feeling of well-being. Swimming, walking and dancing are arguably the most natural, and therefore the most beneficial, forms of movement. Or you might like to take up yoga, which is a good all-rounder for both body and mind.

Let us now consider massage.

The Effects of Massage

Although massage cannot totally replace physical activity, it is in fact similar, in body stimulation terms, to 20 minutes of jogging! Therefore, regular massage (with or without essential oils) is especially beneficial to those who are forced to lead a sedentary lifestyle, perhaps through ill health, advanced age or physical disability. Above all, if carried out with flowing sensitivity rather than in a stiff and mechanical manner, the Tender Loving Care aspect of massage can be the most deeply healing force.

The moment you place your hands on another person, you begin to treat body and mind simultaneously. The nerves awaken immediately, relaying messages to the brain, which then sends out 'reaction' instructions throughout the body.

By improving blood circulation and lymphatic drainage, massage aids the elimination of tissue wastes such as lactic and carbonic acids, which often build up in the muscle fibres, causing muscular aches and pains or stiffness. At the same time, the emotional effects of skilled but gentle massage, especially if heightened by the aroma of essential oils, can be profound. It can sometimes bring about a peaceful yet highly alert state of mind similar to that experienced by meditators. As the tense muscles begin to relax, sometimes pent-up emotions are also freed. Some people experience a light-headed sensation, as if they have had a few glasses of wine; a few fall into a deep sleep! While many people feel tranquil after aromatherapy massage, those who are prone to tiredness and lethargy will often feel much more alive and energetic. This is because aromatherapy massage has a balancing effect on the nervous system as a whole, thus engendering a positive state of mind.

Nothing really beneficial can come about, however, unless there is empathy between giver and receiver. So, if you are giving massage, you need to develop the ability to 'tune in', as it were, to the needs of your partner, allowing your hands to move intuitively to any tender spots in their body and to soothe away the pain. This is largely an innate ability, and although it is naturally well developed in a few people, it is something that most of us can cultivate through concentration. Therefore, when giving massage, try not to talk much; focus your attention on the movement of your hands and the feel of your partner's body. In fact, a flowing, rhythmic massage can be a form of meditation. It can have an hypnotic effect on both giver and receiver.

If you are receiving massage, you need to learn how to accept massage passively and with full awareness; that is, by trusting your partner and 'opening' to the experience. This is difficult to achieve if you constantly chatter and move about. Instead, close your eyes, take a few deep breaths, then breathe out with a sigh and relax into the experience. Then, focus your attention on your partner's touch and enjoy the sensation; allow your body to go heavy and limp. Of course, do speak up if something your partner is doing is hurting, or if you feel cold or uncomfortable in any way. Also, when lying on your front, turn your head from one side to the other if your neck feels stiff.

47

Setting the Scene

The room in which you intend to give massage should have a calm, comfortable atmosphere and be very warm. Chilled muscles contract, causing a release of adrenalin — something you are trying to soothe away in the first place. On the matter of decor, according to colour therapists, the jarring vibrations that emanate from zig-zag patterns or from vivid clashing colours, such as salmon-pink with bright orange, or yellow with scarlet, can affect us even when our eyes are closed. Neutral colours or pastel shades are much more conducive to relaxation. Work in natural daylight if possible or under a soft lamp or candlelight. Harsh overhead lighting will only serve to remind you both of an operating theatre or a visit to the dentist! If you live in a noisy area, you may wish to blot out any background disturbance by playing a tape of specially composed relaxation or meditation music. These tapes are now widely available from 'New Age' outlets or from good music shops. However, do keep the volume very low — your partner's senses will be especially acute. As a final touch, you might like to place a vase of fresh flowers or a potted plant in the room to further enhance the atmosphere.

The Massage Surface

Ideally you will have a purpose-built massage couch; realistically, it is more likely that you will have to work at floor level. In fact, although this will be hard work for the person giving the massage, it is actually better for the recipient because it will be easier for the giver to apply beneficial pressure using much of their own body weight. However, giving a massage will feel like hard work if you have a weak back or poor muscle tone in general. So it is important for you to build up your own stamina and flexibility with a sensible exercise programme first. Gentle stretching and bending exercises are beneficial, especially yoga.

A sleeping bag, strip of foam rubber, thick blankets, a soft rug or a folded double-size duvet on the floor will provide the necessary padding under your partner. Cover this with a sheet or towel(s). A second sheet or bath towel will be needed to cover areas of the body you are not working on, thus preventing your partner from becoming chilled. When giving massage, kneel beside your partner (preferably on a carpeted floor to cushion your knees). Do not attempt to give massage at floor level while standing and bending at the waist. (I have seen this done by beginners on introductory massage courses.) Apart from impeding the all-important flow of the massage, it puts an enormous strain on the lower back.

The Massage Oil

Essential oils are never used neat for massage; they must first be diluted in a good quality vegetable oil. The basic instructions for preparing massage oils are to be found in Chapter 6. However, when choosing an oil for a specific therapeutic effect, first refer to the therapeutic index on page 161, then refer to the essential oil profiles in Chapter 3. But do remember to take into account your partner's aroma preference, perhaps offering a selection of 'possibles', then blending accordingly. Remember, we are often instinctively drawn to the essential oil(s) we need.

When not to Massage

Massage is contra-indicated in the following conditions: fever, inflammation (of skin or joints), thrombosis, phlebitis, varicose veins, skin ulcers, rashes or eruptions, swellings, bruises, sprains, torn muscles and ligaments, broken bones and burns — in short, if it hurts, abandon the movement and move on to another area of the body. It is also generally believed that people with cancer should not be massaged because cancer cells may start to spread to the rest of the body via the lymphatic system. However, recent evidence does not appear to bear this out. Very gentle aromatherapy massage is being used in many British hospitals to help uplift the spirits of cancer patients.

Giving Creative Massage

49

The full-body sequence you are about to learn is based on two massage movements: stroking (*effleurage*) and kneading (*pétrissage*). Although professional aromatherapy massage is much more complex, this simple sequence is excellent for the beginner. Even if your first movements may seem uncertain, you will quickly gain confidence, for there is little to remember. Ideally, you will have a friend or partner with whom to exchange aromatherapy massage. By trying out the techniques on each other, you will begin to develop a sense of how massage should feel — and what feels good to you should also feel good to your partner. The following tips will help you develop your own creative, yet skilful style.

Try to keep the whole of your hands in contact with your partner's body, moulding its contours as if you were sculpting clay.

When you need to apply more oil, try not to break contact with your partner's body. Keep one hand on their back, for instance, or arm, foot or head. Ideally, the whole massage should feel like a continuous flowing movement. To break contact mid-flow can feel most disconcerting to the recipient. However, it is fine to break contact once you have reached a natural break in the sequence, i.e. when you have finished working on the back of the body and you wish your partner to turn over.

Add interest by varying your pressure from very light to very strong. It should be lighter over bony areas such as the shins and knees, but quite firm over large muscles such as those either side of the spine and the buttocks. Generally speaking, a firm touch feels good.

Slow movements are calming, while brisk movements are stimulating.

Work with your whole body, not just your hands and arms. When you are kneading, move gently from side to side in time with your hands. Allow your natural rhythm to come to the fore.

50

To give a good massage you need to be totally relaxed and confident, otherwise your partner will pick up your nervousness.

Do remember that sensitivity combined with the sheer pleasure of giving nurturing massage, no matter how basic, far outweighs a full routine of complicated strokes if they are carried out in a mechanical and impersonal manner.

The Back of the Body

Position your partner on their front, head to one side, arms relaxed at the sides or loosely bent, with the hands at shoulder level. (Some people feel more comfortable with a rolled up towel or cushion under the chest and ankles.) Cover your partner with one or two thick towels to keep him or her warm. If you are working on the floor, kneel with your knees slightly apart. If you are using a massage couch, stand with your feet slightly apart so that you are able to bend at the knees, thus enabling you to lean into the strokes.

Before oiling your hands, move to the right of your partner and place your left hand gently on the back of their neck. Place

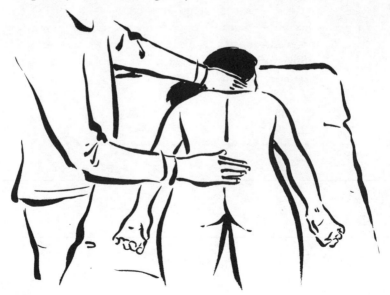

51

Fig. 1: Holding.
Note: Your partner would actually be covered from neck to foot with a towel at this 'tuning in' stage.

your right hand on the base of the spine. Breathe slowly and deeply, allowing yourself to relax. Hold for about half a minute. This has a very calming effect on both parties and, at the same time, enables your partner to become accustomed to your touch (see Fig. 1).

THE LEGS

Pour some previously prepared massage oil into a small dish (never pour oil onto your partner's body, as it can be quite a shock because the oil is usually cooler than body heat). Oil your hands, then rub them together to warm the oil. Remove the towel from the lower half of the body. Starting with the right leg, cross your hands over and, moving both hands together, stroke firmly up the leg from the ankle to the start of the buttocks (see Fig. 2). However, go lightly over the back of the knee. When you reach the top of the leg, fan out your hands and, with a lighter stroke, glide them down either side of the leg. Repeat the movement several times. Knead the calves if you wish. Using each hand alternately, take hold of the flesh with the whole palm of your hand and fingers, pull away from the bone and squeeze as if you were kneading dough. Return to the full-length stroke and carry out once or twice. Repeat the entire sequence on the left leg.

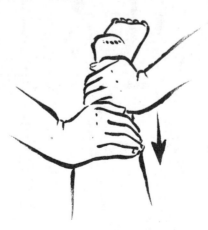

52

Fig. 2: Stroking the back of the leg towards the buttocks.

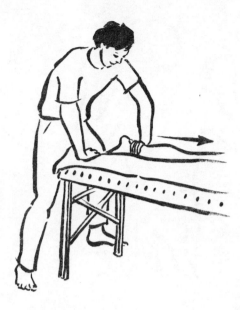

Fig. 3: Stroking both legs together.

Now massage both legs at the same time. Place your right hand across the back of your partner's right ankle, fingers pointing inwards; and your left hand across the back of your partner's left ankle. Leaning into the stroke, slide up the legs and, if your partner is comfortable with this, fan out your hands over the buttocks and glide them lightly back down to the ankles (see Fig. 3). Repeat at least four times. Cover your partner's legs with a towel.

THE BACK, SHOULDERS AND BUTTOCKS
Start with your hands on the lower back, either side of the spine (never apply pressure to the spine itself), your fingers pointing towards the head. Now slide your hands up the back, lean into your hands, using your body weight to apply pressure. When you reach the neck, fan out your hands over the shoulders, then glide them down. As you reach the waist, pull it up gently and return smoothly to the starting point. Repeat several times (see Fig. 4).

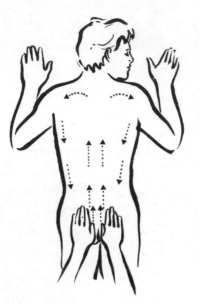
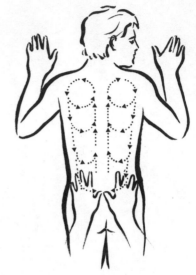

Fig. 4: Long smooth strokes.   *Fig. 5:* Connected circles.

As a slight variation, start with your hands on the lower back as before, and slide firmly up the back. When you reach the shoulders, move your hands in circles over the shoulder blades. Then continue to make connected circles down the back, until you reach the starting position. Repeat several times (see Fig. 5).

Now move your hands to the sides of the body and, starting from the hips or buttocks, begin to knead. Using each hand alternately, take hold of the flesh with the whole palm of your hand and fingers, pull away from the bone and squeeze as if you were kneading dough (see Fig. 6). Keep the whole hand in contact with your partner's body. Work up the sides of the body and across the tops of the arms and shoulders, paying special attention to areas of tightness (tense muscles feel like hard nodules under the skin). When you come to smaller areas (around the shoulder blades, for instance) change to thumbs and two middle fingers, but do not pinch the flesh.

Move to the other side of the body and repeat.

54

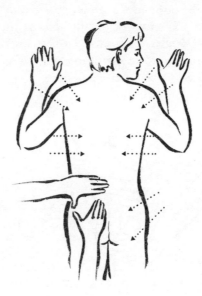

Fig. 6: Kneading.

Finish the back sequence with long smooth strokes from the base to the neck, fanning across the shoulders and down the sides, as before. This time, however, let the stroking become gradually slower and lighter until you are hardly touching your partner at all. Finally, return to the initial holding position. Hold for about half a minute. When you are ready, cover your partner with a towel and ask him or her to turn over. Speak softly, because your partner's senses will be especially acute.

The Front of the Body

Position your partner on their back with a cushion or rolled up towel under the knees to prevent any strain in the lumbar region.

Cover your partner with a towel.

FEET AND LEGS

55

Begin by stroking your partner's right foot. Hold it between your hands and stroke firmly with both hands from the toes towards the body. When you reach the ankles, return your hands to the toes with a light stroke (see Fig. 7). Repeat several times. Then work on the sole of the foot with the thumbs of both hands. Make small circles covering the entire sole (see Fig. 8). Return to the stroking with which you began, then repeat the sequence on the left foot.

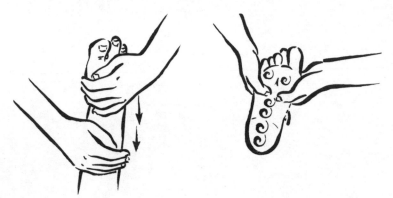

Fig. 7: Stroking the foot.

Fig. 8: Small thumb circles over the sole of the foot.

Now move to a position alongside your partner's right leg. Then as for the backs of the legs, cross and cup your hands over the ankle and glide both hands from one end of the leg to the other. When you reach the top of the thigh, fan out your hands and glide them down the sides (see Fig. 9a and b). Repeat several times, then work on the left leg.

56

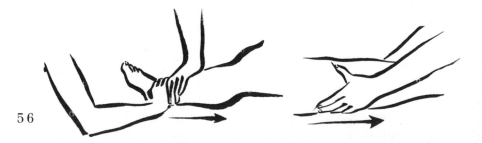

Fig. 9a and b: Stroking the front of the leg.

Cover your partner's legs and feet with a towel before moving to the next stage.

THE ARMS
Starting with the right arm, rest both your hands palms down on your partner's wrist and lower arm. Pressing firmly, glide both hands together up the arm. When you reach the top, separate your hands and glide them back down the full length of the arm and over the hands (see Fig 10a and b). Repeat several times.

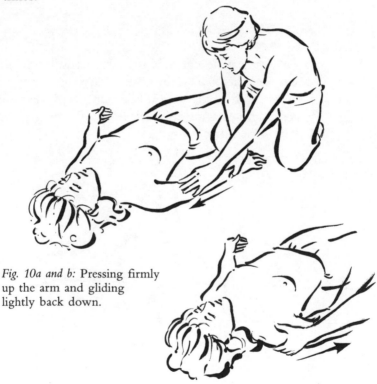

Fig. 10a and b: Pressing firmly up the arm and gliding lightly back down.

Raise your partner's forearm so that it is standing upright with the elbow resting on the floor or table. Then begin massaging the inside of the wrist with the balls of your thumbs. Use your thumbs alternately as you work down the arm to the elbow (see Fig. 11). Repeat several times.

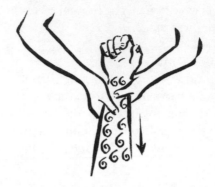

Fig. 11: Thumb circles from the wrist to the elbow.

Bend your partner's arm at the elbow and let the hand dangle down the other side of the neck. Grasp the arm near the elbow between both hands and pull down toward the shoulder joint, alternately squeezing and releasing as you go (see Fig. 12). Repeat several times.

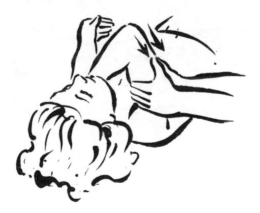

Fig. 12: Squeezing and releasing the upper arm.

58 Return to the sliding movement with which you began, ensuring that you move over the hands and off at the fingertips. Then work on the left arm.

THE ABDOMEN

If your partner agrees, then massage the abdomen. (Some people are apprehensive about having their abdomen massaged.) This is a very sensitive area, so use light pressure.

Move to one side of your partner; let your hands rest very gently over the naval and remain there for a few moments. Begin to massage the whole belly lightly, moving both hands (fingers and palms) clockwise around it, following the coil of the colon. You will find that one hand can complete full circles, but the other will have to break contact each time the hands cross (see Fig. 13). Complete the sequence by allowing your hands to rest lightly over the naval as before.

If your partner is suffering from a great deal of nervous tension, you can massage the solar plexus region or midriff in an anti-clockwise direction (a technique advocated by top aromatherapist Micheline Arcier). Using the right hand and resting the left hand on your partner's arm, gently stroke around the area several times before coming to rest over the naval. Remember to cover your partner with a towel before moving on to the next stage.

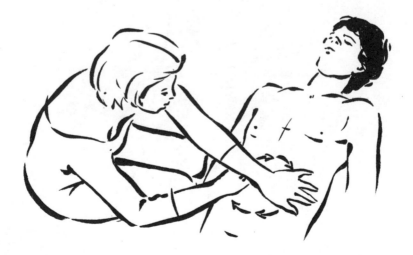

59

Fig. 13: Circling the abdomen.

THE FACE

Before oiling your hands, place them on either side of your partner's head, the heels of the hands covering the forehead, the fingers extending downwards, anchoring the sides of the head. Hold them there for a few moments (see Fig. 14).

Oil your hands. You will only need a tiny amount; if you drench the skin, oil is liable to seep into your partner's eyes. Gently slide your hands over your partner's face, starting from the throat and sweeping up to the chin using the whole surface of your hands. Circle the cheeks, move around the eyes and over the forehead. This is to oil the skin before you begin the main part of the massage (see Fig. 15).

Place the ball of your thumbs at the centre of the forehead between the eyebrows. Slide both thumbs apart and, when you reach the temples, finish with a little circular flourish before gliding off at the hairline. Then start a little higher up, sliding your thumbs apart a strip at a time all the way up to the forehead until you reach the hairline (see Fig. 16).

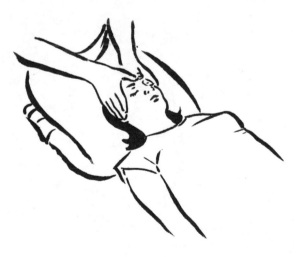

60

Fig. 14: Holding position for face massage.

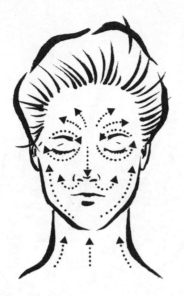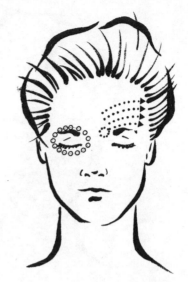

Fig. 15: Oiling the face and neck.   *Fig. 16:* Stroking the forehead and pressure points around the eyes.

Place the ball of your thumbs at the centre between the eyebrows. Press your thumbs down quite firmly (your partner will tell you if it is too hard) and hold for about three seconds. Lift your thumbs and place them a little further along the browbone and repeat the pressure. Repeat at intervals until you reach the outer corners of the eyes (see Fig. 16).

Place your forefingers on the bony ridge *under* the eyes at the inner corners and repeat the pressing movements, a little less heavily this time, until you reach the outer corner (see Fig. 16). Pressure point massage around the eye area helps to release sinus congestion and facial tension. Return to the whole face stroking with which you began and repeat it a few times more before beginning the next stroke.

Using your middle fingers, make tiny circles on the cheeks at either side of the nostrils, then over the upper lip and the chin (see Fig. 17).

61

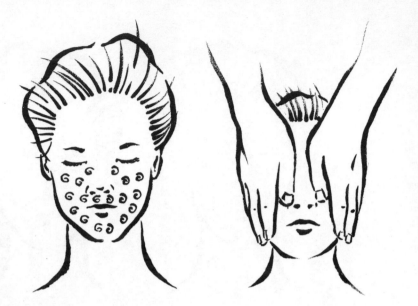

Fig. 17: Using middle fingers to circle the cheeks, upper lip and chin.

Fig. 18: Bathing in darkness.

Now allow your partner to bathe in darkness for a few moments. Place your hands gently over the eyes, the heels of your hands creating the darkness, with the fingers extending down over the temples. Keep them there for about half a minute (see Fig. 18).

Slide your hands to the sides of your partner's head and apply a little pressure to the temples for about 10 seconds before slowly moving to the next stage.

THE NECK

Oil your hands, then gently turn your partner's head to the left. Place your left hand on their forehead, or, if you prefer, support the head by letting it rest in your left hand. Place your right hand on your partner's right shoulder and slide your hand firmly all the way up to the neck. When you reach the base of the skull, use all your fingers and gently circle the area several times to release any muscle tension. Work from the base of the neck upwards to behind the ears (see Fig. 19a and b). Return to the sliding movement and repeat several times before slowly turning your partner's head to the right. Repeat the sequence on the left side.

Gently move your partner's head to the middle so that he or she is lying straight once more. Now give the neck a good stretch. Clasp your hands together at the back of the neck and lift the head a few inches from the massage surface; pull from the base of the skull towards you. Still supporting your partner's head, allow it to come back down gently (see Fig. 20). Repeat several times. Finally, using both hands at the back of the skull, lift your partner's head slowly forward as far as it will comfortably go before allowing it to come gently down (see Fig. 21).

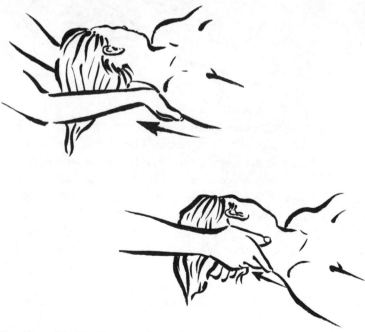

63

Fig. 19a and b: Working on the neck.

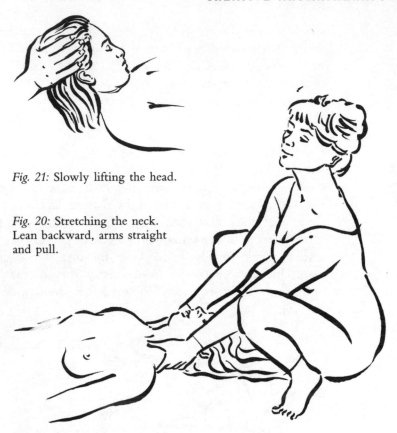

Fig. 21: Slowly lifting the head.

Fig. 20: Stretching the neck.
Lean backward, arms straight
and pull.

THE SCALP

Unless your partner is completely bald there is no need to oil
the scalp. Lift your partner's head and turn it to the left. Using
your fingers, press quite firmly and move fingers *and* scalp over
the bone. Try not to simply slide your fingers through the hair
over the scalp. Work up and down the head covering the entire
area. Repeat on the other side, then move the head back to the
centre. Run your fingers through your partner's hair several
times, allowing your fingers to brush the scalp (see Fig. 22a, b
and c).

64

Finish the entire face, neck and scalp sequence by allowing your
partner to 'bathe in darkness' once again. Move your hands
slowly away.

Fig. 22a, b and c: Working on the scalp, running your fingers through the hair.

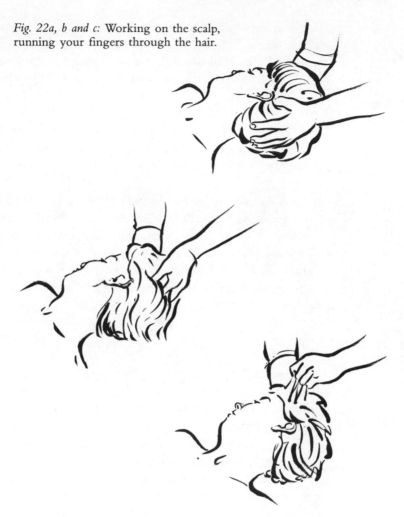

'Feathering'

You might like to conclude with a full-body stroke known as 'feathering'. It is carried out after you have covered your partner from neck to toe with towels. In fact, I often begin and end a massage with feathering, especially if there has only been time to massage one part of the body, the back for instance. Feathering, combined with holding, has a generally balancing effect, engendering in the recipient a sense of connectedness with their whole body.

Begin at the top of the head and 'feather' downwards over the whole body. That is, with hands very relaxed, fingers loosely separated, brush in one long sweeping movement down to the feet. The stroking should be extremely light, barely perceptible to your partner.

On reaching the toes, take your hands back to the head and sweep downwards again. Do this at least a dozen times with rhythmic, flowing movements.

Even if you choose to leave out feathering, complete the entire massage sequence with holding: hold the feet for about half a minute, then the knees, the hands and finally the head and abdomen (place one hand on your partner's forehead, the other lightly on the abdomen). When you are ready, gently move away. Allow your partner to rest for a while and to 'come round' in their own time (see Fig. 23).

Self-Massage

You can also derive a great deal of benefit from massaging the oils into your own skin — though you will, of course, miss out on the deep relaxation aspect of receiving a good massage. The best results are obtained by applying the oils after a warm bath or shower because they will penetrate the skin more readily if it is slightly warm and damp.

The direction of your movements should always be towards the heart to encourage a good flow of blood, and therefore nutrients, to the part being treated. Stroke the skin hand-over-hand in an upward direction. Begin with very light strokes and gradually let them become firmer. Once you have improved the circulation, you can begin to knead the fleshy areas of your body such as the thighs and calves. When you reach the abdomen, gently circle the area in a clockwise direction, thus following the coil of the colon, just as you would when massaging another person. Finish the massage the way you began with hand-over-hand stroking.

However, there is an exception to the 'towards the heart' rule.

66

If you are in an extremely tense state, it can be beneficial to use very light stroking movements in a downward direction (the 'feathering' stroke mentioned earlier), and to massage the solar plexus region (just above the navel) in an anti-clockwise direction. When you feel calmer, continue with the usual massage strokes, but end with feathering.

Let us continue with some other aromatherapeutic techniques.

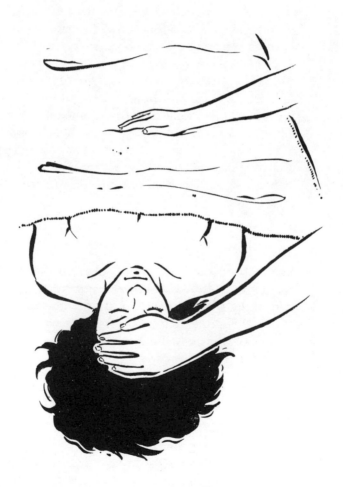

67

Fig. 23: Complete the sequence by holding the forehead and abdomen.

Skin Care

A healthy skin is a reflection of good health in general. Therefore, no amount of external treatment with the finest plant oils will help much if your diet, lifestyle and emotions are out of balance. If you treat your skin from this perspective, the oils will work more efficiently, adding much more than just polish!

Even if you are one of the lucky few, blessed with a trouble-free skin, the use of essential oils and other non-synthetic preparations will help to preserve the suppleness of the skin for as long as possible. Since the aromatic molecules of plant essences penetrate into the deepest layers of the skin (and end up in the bloodstream), they can have a positively profound effect. They act to nourish, tone, detoxify, soothe and generally support the skin's functions.

Essential oils should never be applied neat for skin care, but diluted in a high quality base oil such as almond, extra virgin olive, jojoba or sunflowerseed. The basic instructions for preparing essential oils for skin care are to be found in Chapter 6; here we shall concentrate on how to gain the maximum benefit from their use.

Using Facial Oils

The most effective way to use an aromatherapy facial oil is to apply it as a periodic treatment, either once a week or daily for two weeks with a three to four week interval before resuming again. This prevents the skin from becoming too accustomed to the essences and failing to respond positively to them. The skin likes to be surprised!

There are four ways of applying aromatherapy oils for skin treatments:

1. Apply a fine film just after a bath or shower when your skin is still warm and moist. Do not wipe off any excess for at least 20 minutes — it can take this long for the oils to be absorbed. In fact, unless your skin is very congested, there will be very little, if any, excess oil to remove.

2. Apply as a facial compress to facilitate penetration of the oils (see below).

3. Apply 15–20 minutes after a face pack or facial sauna (see below). The skin needs time to settle down after deep cleansing treatments, otherwise the oils will not be efficiently absorbed.

4. Apply shortly before going for a walk in the open air (preferably the park or unpolluted country air). The combination of oxygen and essential oil is a superb skin rejuvenator.

If you opt for the once a week regime, apply the oils three times a day if possible, though once a day may be enough for some skins.

Instead of using a facial oil you might prefer to 'doctor' an unperfumed commercial cream or lotion (preferably a 'natural' product) with the appropriate oils for your skin type. Stir in 2 or 3 drops of essential oil to every 50 grams of cream or 1 or 2 drops to every 25 ml of lotion and shake well.

Essential oils used in baths and general massage will also help the complexion, whether or not they are applied directly to the face. This is because they reach the bloodstream via the lungs and skin and work systemically, influencing the body as a whole. Very congested skin cannot absorb essential oils efficiently anyway, unless aided by warmth and damp as suggested above, but when used in the bath and in general massage, oils can be more easily absorbed through the softer skin of the abdomen, inner sides of the thighs and upper arms.

If you have an oily complexion, you may be apprehensive about applying oils to your skin. However, the vegetable oil base is mainly a spreading agent; the non-greasy essential oils do most of the work. Any excess oil can be wiped off after about 20 minutes. Unrefined vegetable oils or jojoba wax are recommended as spreading agents because they will not clog the pores. Furthermore, they contain many useful nutrients, such as vitamins A and E, and the essential fatty acids which contribute to skin health.

69

The Facial Sauna

A facial sauna is a deep cleansing treatment which is good for all skin types, but especially for blemished and congested skin.

Put 1 or 2 drops of an essence suitable for your skin type (see page 91) into a bowl containing ½ a litre of steaming water. Cover your whole head with a towel and put it over the steaming bowl so the towel forms a 'tent' to catch the steam. Stay there for up to 5 minutes. Finish this treatment by splashing your face with cool water to remove wastes accumulated on the surface of the skin. Wait 15—20 minutes before applying a moisturiser or an aromatherapy facial oil (recipes in Chapter 6). The skin needs to settle down after a deep cleansing treatment, otherwise the oils will not be efficiently absorbed.

CAUTION:
Saunas must be avoided at all costs if your skin is prone to thread veins. The intense heat will dilate the blood vessels lying under the skin's surface, thus exacerbating the problem.

Saunas should also be avoided if you suffer from asthma; concentrated steam may trigger an attack.

Too many treatments (more than two a week over a period of many months) can cause 'jungle acne' — a disorder brought about by the presence of excess moisture in the skin. If used sensibly though, once a week perhaps, saunas will certainly benefit your skin. It will begin to look and feel revitalized.

A Facial Compress

A warm facial compress opens the pores of the skin, thus enabling the essential oils to penetrate faster and deeper.

Apply an aromatherapy facial oil suitable for your skin type to a thoroughly cleansed skin. You will need a piece of cotton fabric, a clean handkerchief or a face flannel. Cut out 2 holes for your eyes. Briefly immerse the material in a bowl of hand-hot water, then lie down and apply it to your face. Leave it in place for about 5 minutes, then renew it and leave it for a further 5 minutes.

Alternatively, add 2 or 3 drops of essential oil to 1 pint (600 ml) of hand-hot water. Agitate the water to disperse the essences, then immerse the material in the water. Apply to cleansed skin. As in the previous method, leave in place for 5 minutes, then renew and leave for a further 5 minutes.

Face Packs

A weekly face pack, or mask as they are often called, can be applied to the face and neck after ordinary cleansing, or better still, after an aromatic bath or facial sauna while the skin is still warm and moist, and therefore more receptive to whatever you put on it. Face packs are designed to cleanse deeply and balance skin secretions. They are especially good for those times when your skin needs a 'pick-me-up'. (Recipes for face packs are in Chapter 6.)

Dry Skin Brushing

The benefits of this old and well-proven European 'nature cure' technique are amazing. Not only does it condition the skin itself by removing the build up of dead skin cells on the surface, but it also stimulates lymphatic drainage and the elimination of as much as one third of body wastes. According to natural healing principles, these toxins can lead to disease if they are allowed to accumulate in the body. Complaints such as arthritis, cellulite, high blood pressure and even depression have been linked to poor lymphatic drainage. (The lymphatic system is concerned with our immune defences – the production of antibodies against infection – and with the elimination of toxic wastes through the skin, lungs, kidneys and colon.)

In aromatherapy, skin brushing is more commonly used to combat cellulite and, combined with good massage, essential oils and a cleansing diet, it is very effective for this purpose. However, it is also an all-round health aid, suitable for most people, especially the sedentary, the elderly – or the simply lazy! Like massage, dry skin brushing is similar in body stimulation terms to 20 minutes of strenuous exercise. However,

71

be careful if you suffer from a skin disorder such as eczema or psoriasis or if you have any infected or broken skin. Brush where the skin is healthy and avoid any areas where you have bad varicose veins.

How to do it:

You will need a purpose-designed vegetable bristle brush (nylon or animal bristles are, respectively, too soft or too rough) with a long, but detachable handle so that you can reach your back. These are available from many health shops and a few chemists. The brush must always be kept dry but washed in warm soapy water every two weeks. The body needs to be brushed once a day for a few minutes before your morning bath or shower, twice daily if you have cellulite. It is a good idea to take a week's break every month as skin brushing, like many natural detoxification techniques, is more effective if the body does not become too accustomed to it.

Begin at the tips of your shoulders and cover your whole body with long sweeping strokes. Go downwards over the arms, shoulders and upper chest, then upwards over the feet, legs and buttocks to the middle back, excepting the face and nipples, which are too sensitive for this treatment. Always work towards the heart and bring toxins towards the colon. You will need to go over the skin only once or twice. Finally, brush the abdomen (avoiding the genitals), using a clockwise circular motion.

Exfoliation

Dry skin brushing is too harsh for the softer skin of the face, so wet exfoliation is used instead. This will improve the texture of the skin, particularly if you are over 30. Younger skins tend to shed dead skin cells without help, but as we age, the reproduction processes under the skin slow down. New skin cells are formed more slowly and worn-out cells, which are pushed to the surface, tend to stay around in patches.

How to do it:

Moisten a handful of medium ground oatmeal (cornmeal or ground almonds if your skin is dry) and use as a gentle scrub. Rub into all parts of your face and throat. Be especially attentive around the nostrils. Rinse off with warm to cool water. Incidentally, if you are a man who shaves, you may not need to bother with this, as shaving amounts to the same thing. However, you could use the scrub over the smooth areas, the forehead, nose and cheeks from time to time.

Aromatic Baths

Essential oils can be added to your bath simply for pleasure, to aid restful sleep, to help skin disorders, to relieve muscular and other pains or to uplift your spirits. They can be used singly or blended with other essential oils to create an interesting bouquet.

Put 5 to 8 drops of neat essential oil on to the surface of the water *after* you have drawn the bath, then agitate the water to disperse the oil. If you add the essential oil as the water is running, much of the aromatic vapour will have evaporated before you enter the bath. If you have dry skin, you may wish to mix the essence(s) with a few teaspoonfuls of vegetable oil; that is, if you do not mind cleaning a greasy bath afterwards!

For a more soluble bath preparation, mix the usual amount of essential oil into a dessertspoonful of unperfumed liquid soap or a few teaspoonsful of a mild shampoo. Then lie back and relax for at least 20 minutes, luxuriate in the fragrant water and dream!

Foot/Hand Baths

These can be used to ward off chills, for rheumatic or arthritic pain, excessive perspiration, athlete's foot and other skin disorders of the feet or hands such as chilblains, dermatitis or eczema. Put 4 to 6 drops of essential oil (diluted in a few teaspoonsful of vegetable oil if desired) to a bowl of hand-hot water and steep feet (or hands) for about 10 minutes. Dry them thoroughly and massage into the skin a little vegetable oil (or cream) containing a few drops of the same essence(s).

Inhalations

These can be used for colds, 'flu, sinusitis, coughs, catarrh, hay fever and other respiratory disorders. They can also be used to bolster a flagging memory. Essences of basil, rosemary and peppermint are known to have 'cephalic' properties — they stimulate clarity of thought. The simplest method is to put 5 to 10 drops of essential oil on to a handkerchief and inhale as required. Drops of the appropriate essential oil can also be sprinkled on to your pillow to ease nasal congestion and to aid restful sleep. If you do not wish to put essential oils directly on to the pillow, put them on a clean handkerchief and leave nearby.

A more powerful decongestant is the steam inhalation — *but avoid this if you suffer from asthma.* Steam inhalations can be employed to help other respiratory problems such as those mentioned above, or, as already mentioned, they can be used as a deep cleansing facial (see page 74).

Pour about ½ a litre of near-boiling water into a bowl and add 2 to 4 drops of essential oil. The quantity depends on the strength of the essence. Peppermint, for example, is extremely powerful, whereas sandalwood is very mild. Inhale the vapours for about 5 minutes, but no longer than 10. To trap the aromatic steam more efficiently, drape a towel over your head and the bowl to form a 'tent', as with the facial sauna.

You can enjoy steam inhalations 2 or 3 times a day over a short period, if you are suffering from a cold or the 'flu, for example.

Compresses

74

A compress is a valuable way of treating muscular pain, sprains and bruises as well as reducing pain and congestion in internal organs. However, it is vital to know when to apply a cold compress and when to apply a warm compress:

Cold: These are for recent injuries such as sprains, bruises, swellings, inflammation and headaches.

Warm: These are for old injuries, muscular pain, toothache, menstrual cramp, cystitis, boils and abscesses.

To make a warm compress, add about 6 drops of essential oil to a bowl of water containing about ½ a litre of water, as hot as you can comfortably bear. Place a small towel or a piece of lint or cotton fabric on top of the water. Wring out the excess and place the fabric over the area to be treated. Cover this with a piece of clingfilm, then lightly bandage in place if necessary (for an ankle or knee for example). Leave the compress in place until it has cooled to body temperature; renew at intervals as required.

For a cold compress, use exactly the same method, but with very cold (preferably icy) water. Leave in place until it warms to body heat and renew as required.

Using Undiluted Essential Oils

Eucalyptus, tea tree or lavender oil can be applied neat as an antiseptic for cuts, grazes, wounds, insect bites and stings, and so forth. My own preference is for lavender because it is less likely to irritate the skin. Moreover, undiluted lavender essence is remarkably effective for athlete's foot.

Perfumes

Perfuming Rooms

Perfuming a room with essential oils creates an interesting ambience which can have a subtle effect on the mood of its occupants. The most effective way to perfume a room is to use a purpose-designed essential oil burner/vaporizer or an electric fragrancer. These are now widely available from health shops and essential oil suppliers. A few drops is all you will need for at least half an hour of fragrance (see Chapter 8). Alternatively, you may prefer to buy a purpose-designed fragrance ring: a ceramic or cardboard disc that balances over the top of the light bulb. The essences are dropped on the ring and the warmth from the bulb releases the aromatic vapour.

You could also put a few drops of essential oil in a saucer of water and place on top of a radiator, or put the drops in a purpose-designed radiator humidifier.

Another method of room fragrancing is to spray a few drops of essential oil around the home using either an atomiser or simple plant spray. Add about 5 drops of your favourite essence(s) to 142 ml of water and shake well before use. However, the effect is short-lived compared with the previous methods.

Room sprays can also be used to pleasantly fumigate the home to help prevent the spread of infection during epidemics. For this purpose, use up to 15 drops of oil in the same quantity of water. The following essences are the most powerful against airborne bacteria: pine, peppermint, lavender, lemon, rosemary, cloves, cinnamon, eucalyptus and tea tree. The last two oils are also credited with anti-viral properties as well, and are useful should a member of the family be stricken with 'flu.

Skin Perfumes

As we shall discover in Chapter 7, essential oils can be used either alone or blended with other essences to make delightful perfumes. They may be used purely for pleasure or to back up the healing potential of other aromatherapy treatments — particularly for stress-related problems. For the occasional attack of anxiety or depression, a blend of carefully selected essences will uplift your spirits. When anxiety or depression becomes a way of life, however, it would be advisable to seek the help of a professional counsellor, aromatherapist or other holistic health practitioner.

5 · The Alchemist's Larder

The essential oils listed in Chapter 3 are the oils I tend to use most often. However, such a selection would be extremely costly if you were to buy them all at once. Indeed, my own aromatic store of around 50 essences has developed over a number of years. If you wish to begin experimenting with essential oils, about half a dozen carefully chosen essences will be sufficient — that is, until the aromatic quest beckons you further into the ethereal realms!

Although aroma preference may be vital to the efficacy of the finished product, when choosing oils for creative aromatherapy, do not be put off by an essence that does not immediately smell interesting. You may discover that it smells wonderful when used in tiny quantities and blended with other essences. Vetiver and patchouli are good examples. On first acquaintance with these heavy, earthy and definitely Eastern fragrances, you may wonder how they could ever be perceived as beautiful. Yet blend either of these strangers with larger quantities of the more familiar fragrances of bergamot, mandarin, orange, lavender or perhaps geranium, and there is a successful marriage of opposites. The brighter citrus or floral essences act to awaken the heavy lingerers, elevating the aroma to a higher plane. At the same time, the powerful embrace of vetiver or patchouli serves to hold back the more volatile essences whose presence would otherwise be relatively fleeting (see Chapter 7).

Ideally, your initial selection of oils will include a representative from each of the aroma families as listed below:

Balsamic or resinous — frankincense, myrrh.
  Hint: Myrrh tends to harden into a sticky gum, so it is difficult to work with. You may need to warm the bottle in

a cup of hot water before use. It has to be said that the aroma does not appeal to many people, though it can be interesting as a background note in blends.

Citrus — bergamot, grapefruit, lemon, lime, mandarin, orange.
Hint: Bergamot is perhaps the most versatile, blending well with many other oils. It also has a longer shelf-life than the other citrus essences.

Earthy — patchouli, vetiver.

Floral — geranium, lavender, neroli (orange blossom), rose otto, ylang ylang.
Hint: If you like the aroma of neroli, but find the price prohibitive, try the much cheaper, similar-smelling petit-grain which is distilled from the leaves of the orange tree. The aroma is much less refined than that of its floral sister, but acceptable as a background note in blends. Alas, there is nothing to match the unique aroma of the costly rose otto. Indeed, even the most expensive synthetic rose oils (and some are only marginally cheaper than the actual essence) need to contain a tiny amount of the real thing, for it is impossible to re-create the true fragrance of this exquisite oil.

Herbal — basil, camomile, clary sage, marjoram, peppermint, rosemary.

Medicinal — eucalyptus, tea tree.

Pine-like — cypress, juniper, pine.

Spicy — black pepper, cardomom, cinnamon bark, clove, coriander, ginger.
CAUTION: Cinnamon bark and clove should only be used to perfume rooms, for these essences can cause skin irritation.

Woody — cedarwood, sandalwood.

You could group the woody, pine-like and medicinal families together (partly because they are from trees and also because they tend to blend well with each other, albeit in a rather conservative way!)

Having purchased your precious essential oils, it is vital to store them in a cool dark place, otherwise they will rapidly deteriorate, losing not only their original clarity of fragrance, but also much of their therapeutic potency (see *Caring for your*

Oils, page 29). Remember too that the 'bouquet' of an essential oil, like wine, will vary from year to year according to changes in climatic conditions. So do not expect the same type of lavender oil, for instance, that is, the same named botanical species — good quality oils are always listed according to botanical species — to smell exactly the same each harvest, especially if produced in a different country from the last batch you may have purchased. Plants absorb something of the atmosphere of the place in which they are grown, and this contributes to the character of the essential oil.

Base Oils

Essential oils intended for aromatherapy massage need to be diluted in a fine quality vegetable oil such as almond, apricot kernel or sunflower seed — preferably unrefined or 'cold-pressed'. If an oil is not labelled as such, it is certain to be a refined product extracted by high pressure, intense heat and possibly even chemical solvents.

Unlike refined oils such as soya or corn, unrefined vegetable oils are rich in fat-soluble nutrients and essential fatty acids which can easily be absorbed through the skin and utilized by the body. Even without the addition of essential oils, these vegetable oils are health treatments in themselves. Extra virgin olive oil, for example, soothes inflamed skin and is helpful as a massage oil for arthritic complaints.

However, never use mineral oil (baby oil), as this is derived from petroleum. Not only does mineral oil lack the health-giving properties of unrefined vegetable oil, but according to many health experts, mineral oil applied to the skin (or taken internally) makes fat-soluble nutrients such as vitamins A and E leach from the body. Moreover, it tends to clog the pores of the skin, thus contributing to the development of blackheads and pimples. Above all, the use of synthetic oil of any nature (and that includes synthetic essential oils) is antithetical to the philosophy of aromatherapy.

Most aromatherapists favour bland base oils such as almond

or grapeseed because such oils do not impart their own aroma to the fragrant blends. However, to my nose, the faintly nutty odour of unrefined vegetable oil (or its pungency, if olive oil) does, in fact, blend harmoniously with the aromas of essential oils. For a more economical, less nutty or pungent blend, you could mix a refined oil such as grapeseed with an equal quantity (or less) of an unrefined oil such as extra virgin olive, sunflower seed or sesame. However, if you use sesame oil, ensure that it is the light-coloured oil from the *raw* seed. The dark, strongly flavoured oil obtained from toasted sesame seed does not blend harmoniously with essential oils — unless you relish smelling like a Chinese stir-fry!

For a facial oil, jojoba (pronounced *ho ho ba*) is one of the lightest to use, either alone or blended with other vegetable oils. It can even be used on oily or acneous skin. In fact, jojoba is a liquid wax rather than a true vegetable oil. It is extracted from a small evergreen plant native to the desert regions of South America.

Other useful oils include macadamia nut, hazelnut and avocado. The latter oil is very rich, yet it has a fine texture which the skin can easily absorb. It makes an excellent facial oil for dry or mature skin, though you may prefer to dilute it with a lighter vegetable oil such as almond or apricot kernel.

Grapeseed oil and also unrefined or cold-pressed vegetable oils are available from health shops and some supermarkets. The speciality oils such as avocado, peach kernel and jojoba are easier to obtain by mail order from most essential oil suppliers (see the addresses on pages 158–60).

Shelf-Life

If kept in the fridge, most cold-pressed oils will keep for up to nine months, but do check the best-before date. Incidentally, when kept in very cool temperatures, unrefined oils tend to go cloudy — a good sign indicating that the oil is of a high quality. Jojoba, on the other hand, can be stored at room temperature (it solidifies in cool temperatures), and due to its unusual anti-bacterial properties, tends not to turn rancid.

Other Intriguing Bounties

If you intend to take 'kitchen alchemy' seriously, then you will also need a supply of all or some of the following ingredients:

Bach Flower Remedies (optional) — the Remedies act to broaden the psychotherapeutic effects of essential oils (see Chapter 9). They are obtainable from many health shops and a few chemists or directly from the Bach Centre (see the mail order address in the Appendix).

Beeswax — available from herbal suppliers, craft shops or from some bee keepers. A healing emulsifier for skin creams. Try to obtain yellow beeswax rather than the refined white version.

Brewer's yeast powder — makes a nourishing face pack for oily, sallow or fatigued skin.

Cocoa butter — available from herbal suppliers. A wonderful skin-softening agent.

Distilled water — available from most chemists.

Fine oatmeal or ground almonds — nourishing binding agents for face packs. Medium ground oatmeal makes a good facial scrub for removing the build up of dead skin cells.

Floral waters — orange flower water, rosewater, witch hazel. These are available from most chemists or herbal suppliers.

Fractionated coconut oil (labelled 'Light Coconut') — a highly refined oil which makes a good base for home-made perfumes. Unlike whole coconut oil, which is solid at room temperature, light coconut is liquid. Purists may prefer to use unrefined jojoba as a perfume base.

Fuller's Earth — a healing clay, available in powdered form from most chemists. Makes a stimulating face pack for oily skin and acne.

Live, full-fat natural yoghurt — makes a balancing face pack for most skins, except the very dry.

Organic cider vinegar — restores the acid/alkali balance of the skin.

Raw honey — that which has not been pasturized, pressure filtered or blended with other honeys. Available direct from some bee keepers or from health shops. Honey heals and moisturizes the skin.

Equipment

You will also need an ample supply of screw-top bottles and jars — these are available in various sizes from most chemists and essential oil suppliers, or from specialist shops selling home-made cosmetic materials and herbs. You can, of course, re-cycle any suitable glass containers, but do not use plastic bottles and jars. Essential oils tend to react with plastic, especially if in contact with the substance for any length of time.

Other useful items include:

Coffee filter papers for filtering skin/hair tonics and perfumes.

Enamel or stainless steel double boiler *or* a heat-resistant glass or pottery bowl which will fit over a small saucepan of simmering water.

Essential oil burner or electric fragrancer (available from health shops and essential oil suppliers).

Eye dropper or pipette.

Glass measuring jug and small funnel.

Heat-proof bowls.

Kitchen grater suitable for grating beeswax.

Nylon sieve or piece of muslin for straining herbal preparations.

Palette knife, teaspoon, desertspoon, tablespoon.

Plastic 5 ml medicine spoon for measuring small quantities of base oil (available from chemists).

Rotary whisk *or* an electric whisk with a choice of settings. (Do not use a blender for mixing creams and ointments; the high speed causes the mixture to separate or curdle.)

Self-adhesive labels — for labelling your aromatic concoctions.

Set of kitchen scales capable of measuring small quantities.

Vodka — for making your own vanilla extract.

Weights And Measures

For the benefit of American readers, the following conversion table should be helpful:

Liquid Measure (Dry if appropriate.)
   1 teaspoon (t) = 5 ml
   3 teaspoons = 1 tablespoon (T) = 15 ml
   2 tablespoons = 30 ml = 1 fluid oz
   1 cup = 8 fl oz = 0.24 litre (240 ml)
   2 cups = 1 pint = 0.47 litre
   1 pint (29 cubic inches) = 0.47 litre
   4 cups = 1 quart = 0.95 litre
   1 quart = 58 cubic inches = 0.95 litre

Weight
   1 oz = 28.35 g
   1 lb = 453.59 g
   1 lb = 0.45 kg

6 · Apprenticed to Alchemy

This part of the book is devoted to the basic principles of blending vegetable oils, essences and other natural substances for healing purposes as well as for the sheer joy of creative aromatherapy.

Mixing Massage Oils

First choose the essential oil(s) to suit your physical and/or emotional needs, referring to the Therapeutic Index on page 161 and the information in Chapter 3. (If you wish to prepare a facial oil suitable for your skin type, see page 91.)

Essential oils need to be diluted at a rate of ½ to 3 per cent (see Easy Measures below) depending on the person's skin, the strength of the essential oil and the condition for which it is being applied. The lowest concentrations (½ to 1 per cent) are best for facial oils and for those with sensitive skin. If your skin is sensitive, it is best to start with the ½ per cent concentration and, if this causes no irritation, increase to 1 per cent. For a body oil, gradually build up to 2 per cent. In practice, I rarely use concentrations above 2½ per cent for massage (even for those with 'normal' skin). However, 3 per cent concentrations of certain oils can be most helpful when there is a great deal of muscular tension.

CAUTION:

A few oils are very strong and should always be used in concentrations no greater than ½ to 1 per cent. These include basil, camomile, fennel, ginger, lemongrass and melissa.

I tend also to be wary of black pepper, citrus oils, geranium and ylang ylang. These are best used at a concentration no greater than 2 per cent for body massage, for these too can irritate sensitive skins in higher concentrations.

Essences of rose otto and neroli have a very high odour intensity, which means a tiny amount will go a long way. So you will rarely need more than ½ to 1 per cent of these oils in blends.

Easy Measures

If you intend to mix only enough oil for a single massage, use a 5 ml plastic medicine spoon to measure the base or carrier oil. Ordinary teaspoons generally hold less than 5 ml.

Facial Oils

For a ½ per cent concentration add 1 drop of essential oil to every 2 teaspoonsful of base oil. For a 1 per cent concentration, add 1 drop of essential oil to each teaspoonful of base oil. For a 2 per cent concentration, add 2 drops of essential oil to each teaspoonful of base oil. However, do not exceed a 2 per cent concentration when preparing facial oils.

Body Oils

For a 2 or 3 per cent concentration, add two or three drops of essential oil to each teaspoonful of base oil.

For larger quantities of massage oil to be stored in dark glass bottles, fill a 50 ml bottle with a base oil, then add the required amount of essential oil. For a ½ per cent concentration, add 5 drops to 50 ml of base oil. For a 1 per cent concentration in the same amount of base oil, add 10 drops of essential oil; for a 2 per cent concentration, add 20 drops, and for a 3 per cent concentration, add 30 drops. Store in a cool dark place, but use within 2 to 3 months.

Talk Kindly to your Oils!

A phenomenon which never ceases to amaze is the fact that no two people can blend an identical-smelling aromatherapy oil, even though they may use exactly the same blend of oils in exactly the same quantities from the same bottles. Believe it or not, the oil will always take on an aspect of the person's mood or personality. A massage oil or perfume blended whilst you are feeling depressed, angry, nervous or whatever, will not smell right, no matter how beautiful the ingredients. It may smell rather 'flat', 'murky' or somewhat harsh.

However, it is also true that blending aromatics can have a very definite and positive effect on mood, like listening to uplifting music. So if your blends do not appear to be working, stay with the oils for a while longer and you may pass over the threshold into the realm of fragrant harmony. At other times, you may need to abandon any attempt at blending until you have managed to brush away the cobwebs. So try to discover your own source of harmony and inspiration. Perhaps you need to commune with nature — a walk in the park or the countryside might help. Or maybe you are inspirited by animals, certain people, places or things — a beautiful crystal, sculpture or painting, for instance. The key may also be found in music, poetry or a favourite book — a few special words may open the gates. Equally, you may be inspired by strenuous physical activity — swimming, running, hill walking — even weight training or boxing if that is your leaning!

Always, a harmonious blend will mysteriously retain the blender's aromatic signature, the essence of their personality. A flamboyant extrovert, for instance, will magically bestow a note of warmth and colour to blends, even when using rather solemn essences such as cypress, myrrh, pine and juniper. A sweet-natured, timid soul will somehow tone down the earthy or spicy oils such as patchouli, vetiver or ginger. But do not take my word for it; get together with a group of 3 or 4 friends — preferably of widely differing personalities — then carry out the following experiment.

You will need 3 or 4 clean bottles of equal capacity (10 ml

is a good size for this experiment), any base oil and 3 different essential oils with *accurate* dropper caps (all good essential oil suppliers provide graduated dropper caps with their oils). As a suggestion, we shall use lavender, geranium and patchouli.

Method:
Each person in turn should carry out the experiment exactly as follows: fill a bottle with vegetable oil, add 1 drop of patchouli, 2 drops of lavender and 1 drop of geranium, and shake well. Hold the bottle for at least 5 minutes in order for the oil to become imbibed with your personal vibes. Once everyone has completed the task, compare aromas — you will not be disappointed!

Essential Oils for Different Skin Types
To obtain the best results from essential oil skin treatments, read the skin care information in Chapter 3.

Ageing Skin: Frankincense, lavender, myrrh, neroli, rose, sandalwood.

Combination Skin: Camomile, geranium, lavender, rose.

Dehydrated Skin: Camomile, geranium, lavender, rose.

Dry Skin: Camomile, lavender, neroli, rose, sandalwood.

'Normal' Skin: Camomile, geranium, lavender, neroli, rose.

Oily Skin/Acne: Bergamot (but only if Bergamot FCF — see Chapter 3), cypress, eucalyptus, frankincense, geranium, juniper, lavender, lemon, patchouli, pine, rosemary, tea tree.

Puffy Skin (water-logged): cypress, geranium, juniper, lavender, patchouli.

87

Sensitive Skin: Try ½ per cent concentrations of camomile, lavender or rose.

Thread Veins: Camomile, cypress, lemon, rose.

Recipes

Most of the aromatic recipes in this book are 'open-ended', that is to say, there is a choice of essential oils (and other ingredients) to complete the finished product. Your choice will always depend upon your aroma preference, as well as the therapeutic properties of the oils. This will encourage you to experiment and to trust your own instincts.

BALANCING FACIAL OIL

This oil is suitable for most skins, except the very sensitive.

10 ml jojoba oil
20 ml almond oil
4 drops of lavender
2 drops of geranium

Alternative Essences:
Camomile, neroli, rose otto. Remember that these 3 essences have a strong aroma, so you may need fewer than 6 drops of essential oil in the recipe. Let your nose be your guide.

Alternative Base Oils:
Almond, apricot kernel, extra virgin olive, hazelnut, peach kernel, sesame, sunflower seed.

FOR ACNEOUS SKIN

30 ml jojoba oil
2 drops of tea tree
2 drops of patchouli
2 drops of lavender

88

Alternative Essences:
Cypress, eucalyptus, juniper, rosemary.

FOR DRY SKIN

10 ml avocado oil
20 ml apricot kernel oil
4 drops of sandalwood
1 drop of rose otto

Alternative Essences:
Refer to the skin care guide (page 91).

Alternative Base Oils:
Almond, extra virgin olive, hazelnut, macadamia nut.

FOR INFLAMED SKIN

This oil will help soothe eczema, psoriasis, dermatitis and so
forth.

30 ml extra virgin olive oil
Contents of 4 evening primrose oil capsules
2 drops of camomile
4 drops of lavender

Alternative Essence:
Rose otto (no more than 2 drops).

Alternative Base Oils:
Calendula, hypericum, macadamia. Calendula and hypericum
are infused oils, that is to say, they are obtained by maceration —
plant material is seeped in a vegetable oil such as almond and
placed in sunlight for a long period, until the oil becomes
saturated with the therapeutic properties of the plant. Both
calendula and hypericum oils are soothing to inflamed skin,
though hypericum also helps to. alleviate muscular and
rheumatic pain. These oils are available from herbal suppliers,
or you could make your own (see page 99).

FOR MATURE SKIN

20 ml avocado oil
15 ml jojoba oil
Contents of 1 vitamin E capsule
1 or 2 drops of rose otto
2 drops of frankincense
1 drop of sandalwood

Alternative Essences:
Lavender, myrrh, neroli.

Alternative Base Oils:
Almond, extra virgin olive, jojoba, macadamia nut; contents of 2 evening primrose oil capsules.

FOR OILY SKIN

30 ml jojoba oil
4 drops of juniper
1 drop of bergamot
1 drop of lavender

Alternative Essences:
Refer to the skin care guide (page 91).

FOR SENSITIVE SKIN

30 ml almond oil
3 drops of camomile

Alternative Essences:
Neroli, rose otto (1 drop of each or 2 drops of just 1 essence will be sufficient as these essences are highly odoriferous).

Alternative Base Oils:
Apricot kernel, jojoba or peach kernel.

FOR ACHING MUSCLES

25 ml grapeseed oil
25 ml extra virgin olive oil
10 drops of lavender
10 drops of marjoram
5–10 drops of bergamot

Alternative Essences:
You could use 7 drops of camomile to replace the marjoram (camomile is very strong and should be used in lower concentrations), and/or replace the lavender with the same amount of juniper or rosemary. Other suitable essences include black pepper, coriander, cypress, eucalyptus, ginger, pine and tea tree.

Alternative Base Oils:
Hypericum mixed 50/50 with a cheaper base oil of your choice.

RELAXING MASSAGE OIL

25 ml grapeseed oil
25 ml sunflower seed oil
4 drops of clary sage
4 drops of lavender
6 drops of ylang ylang
6 drops of cedarwood

Alternative Essences:
You could replace clary sage with the same quantity of geranium or bergamot. Instead of cedarwood, you could try 3 drops of vetiver *or* 3 drops of patchouli (these two essences have a very tenacious aroma and will overpower the blend if used in greater quantities). Other suitable essences include neroli, rose otto and sandalwood.

Alternative Base Oils:
Any combination.

Cellulite

Cellulite is a peculiarly female problem in which the hormone oestrogen is believed to play a part. It is characterized by unsightly lumps and bumps which collect in the thighs, buttocks, hips and sometimes the upper arms. If the area is pinched, the skin puckers and ripples and does not spring immediately back into place. The affected areas look like orange-peel and are cold to the touch. This is because the underlying tissue is saturated with water and stagnant wastes (unlike ordinary fat).

MASSAGE OIL TO HELP CELLULITE

25 ml almond oil
25 ml extra virgin olive oil
15 drops of juniper
6 drops of orange
4 drops of patchouli

Alternative Essences:
Black pepper, cedarwood, cypress, geranium, lavender, lemon, lime, mandarin, rosemary.

Alternative Base Oils:
Grapeseed, sesame, sunflower seed.

How to use:
Massage the oil into cellulite-laden areas twice daily, using quite vigorous hand-over-hand stroking and kneading — but be careful not to bruise the skin. Use the same essences in the bath to reinforce the effect.

92

Important:
Best results are obtained by changing the recipe every so often, otherwise the body may fail to respond if the same essential oil (or blend) is used for longer than 3 to 4 weeks continuously.

In order to successfully treat cellulite, the oil needs to be used in conjunction with dry skin brushing (see page 75) and a sensible diet consisting of plenty of raw fruit and vegetables and copious amounts of spring water to flush out toxins. Unfortunately there is not enough space in this book to discuss the dietary approach in detail, so I suggest you obtain a copy of Liz Hodgkinson's excellent little book listed in the Bibliography.

Oils for the Hair and Scalp

The finest oil to use for the hair is extra virgin olive. The oil is known to strengthen the hair shafts, thus giving the hair body and shine. In fact, a dessertspoonful of the uncooked oil should also be added to your food daily, for it is rich in fat-soluble vitamins and essential fatty acids, which are extremely beneficial to both hair and skin.

DEEP CONDITIONING TREATMENT FOR DRY OR DAMAGED HAIR

50 ml extra virgin olive oil
10 drops of rosemary
10 drops of lavender

Alternative Essences:
Camomile, geranium, patchouli, sandalwood, ylang ylang.

Additional Ingredient:
A free-range egg yolk beaten into the oils will add to the conditioning treatment. This is especially helpful if your hair is prone to split ends and/or dandruff.

How to use:
Apply to *wet* hair (otherwise it will be difficult to shampoo out); cover your head with a towel and leave on for 15 to 30 minutes before shampooing. Use as a weekly conditioning treatment.

93

TREATMENT FOR HEAD LICE

75 ml of any vegetable oil
15 drops of lavender
5 drops of geranium
5 drops of eucalyptus

Method:
Funnel the vegetable oil into a bottle, add the essential oils and shake well.

Alternative Essences:
Rosemary, tea tree.

How to use:
Apply the essential oil treatment to wet hair (otherwise it will be difficult to shampoo out the oil). Massage well into the scalp to reach the hair roots. Pay particular attention to the areas around the ears and nape of the neck where the lice breed. Leave on for at least an hour, then shampoo thoroughly. Remove the eggs (nits) with a regulation fine-toothed comb. Repeat twice at three-day intervals.

Sunscreen Oils

The most effective natural sunscreens are avocado, almond, sesame, coconut and extra virgin olive oil, but they are not as protective as the high factor commercial preparations available. If your skin burns easily, it may be best to stay out of the sun or use a commercial sun-block preparation.

The sun increases the skin's ability to absorb essential oils, so the concentration of essences in these two recipes is very low. The oils will screen out, on average, 20 per cent of the sun's rays. However, in order to preserve your skin and prevent the possible development of skin cancer, please do not sunbathe between 12 noon and 3.30 p.m. In fact, according to naturopaths (and yogis) the morning rays are the most beneficial to health.

Either of the blends given below can also be used as an after sun soother. If you are using them for this purpose, you may wish to increase the amount of essential oils to about 20 drops.

RICH BLEND

20 ml extra virgin olive oil
20 ml avocado oil
10 ml wheatgerm oil
4 drops of sandalwood

LIGHT BLEND

30 ml coconut oil
20 ml sesame oil
2 drops of lavender
2 drops of camomile

Alternative Essences:
Eucalyptus, tea tree.

Infused Oils

Making your own infused or herbal oils is not only fun, it also ensures the quality of the product, especially if you gather wild plants or use organically grown herbs from your own garden. By macerating plant material in a high quality vegetable oil such as almond or olive, you will obtain a solution of the essential oil in the vegetable oil base, and this can be used undiluted as a massage oil, or if strong enough, mixed 50/50 with a further quantity of vegetable oil. The diluted version is best for children and for those with sensitive skin. You can also add a few drops of essential oil to herbal oils at the rate of about ½ to 1 per cent (see page 89).

95

You can use almost any herb, for example camomile, clary sage, lavender, lemon balm, mint or rosemary. Two of the most useful herbal oils are pot marigold (*calendula officinalis*) and St John's wort (*hypericum perforatum*). Marigold oil is helpful for inflammation of the skin, bruising, muscle strain, period pain, athlete's foot and ringworm. St John's wort oil is a beautiful ruby red and, like marigold, is anti–inflammatory. It can be used externally to ease fibrositis, sciatica and rheumatic pain.

Method:
Pick the healthiest looking flowers and/or leaves on a warm sunny day, after the dew has evaporated. This is the time when the essential oil is at its 'highest' (with the exception of night–scented flowers such as jasmine). You will need about 4 oz (60 g) of plant material to 1 pint (600 ml) of oil. Bruise the herbs by placing on a wooden chopping board and crushing with a rolling pin or a wooden mallet. Half fill a large glass jar with the plant material, then cover with oil. Ensure that the jar is equipped with a tight-fitting lid, then give a really good shake. Place the jar outside in the sun (or in a sunny window) for 2 to 4 weeks — weather permitting — but bring indoors at night. Remember to shake the jar hard whenever you pass by. When ready, press the mixture through muslin or a nylon sieve, then bottle it. If there is a separation of oil and herbal liquid (the oil will float on top), simply decant the oil into another bottle. If stored in a cool dark place, your herbal oils will keep for about a year — from one harvest to the next.

Making Skin Creams and Ointments

Home-made skin creams and ointments are richer and heavier than super-light commercial products, but they are extremely effective and economical. Moreover, beeswax and the finest quality vegetable oils will not clog the pores.

Many books on home-made cosmetics suggest the use of rather dubious substances such as mineral oil (see page 83), alcohol (including surgical spirit), lard (imagine!), borax and glycerin. Although a naturally occurring substance found on alkaline lake shores, borax can be too drying for some skins. Glycerin is a by-product of soap manufacture and has always been regarded as a superb humectant, attracting moisture from the air and thus giving the skin a soft dewy appearance. However, according to Virginia Castleton (the American author and expert on health and skin care), studies have shown that glycerin also attracts moisture from within the outer layers of the skin. This can easily evaporate, leaving the skin taut and parchment-like. The skin then becomes 'hooked', craving regular fixes in order to feel comfortable. As many commercial moisturisers contain glycerin and other similarly acting substances such as glycol, sodium pyrrolidone, propylene or carboxylic acid, at least half the female population in Western society (and some of the men) must be moisturizer 'junkies'!

The following recipe makes a fairly soft cream which will harden slightly if kept in the fridge (to halt the formation of mould), but nevertheless melts on contact with the skin. You will need only a tiny amount, so do not be tempted to make too much — unless you intend sharing the cream with your friends. If kept in a cool place, it should keep for up to 4 months.

BASIC SKIN CREAM

15 g beeswax (grated)
50 ml jojoba oil
70 ml almond oil
30 ml distilled water
6—8 drops of essential oil (see skin care oils, page 91)

Method:
1. Melt the beeswax with the oil in the top of an enamel double boiler or heat-proof basin over a saucepan of simmering water (the *bain marie* method).
2. Meanwhile, heat the distilled water in another basin over a saucepan of simmering water until it has warmed. There is no need to be too precise about temperature, but blood heat is about right.
3. Begin to add the warm distilled water, drop by drop at first, to the oil and wax, beating with a rotary whisk or an electric food mixer set at medium speed.

4. After you have mixed about 2 teaspoonsful of the water into the oil and wax, remove from the heat and continue adding the water a little at a time until you have incorporated every drop.

5. As soon as the mixture begins to thicken, stir in the essential oil.

6. Divide the mixture into little sterilized glass pots, cover tightly and label.

Alternative Ingredients:

You may prefer to use a floral water instead of distilled water. Witch hazel is a gentle antiseptic, astringent liquid, having a tightening effect on the skin. Rosewater and orange flower water impart their own subtle scent to creams. They also act as gentle toners. Rosewater is suitable for all skin types, especially skin that is prone to thread veins. Orange flower water is especially helpful for dry skins.

You can experiment with other vegetable oils in the blend (hazelnut, avocado, sunflower seed, apricot kernel and so forth) as long as they add up to 120 ml in all. Cocoa butter (used in the anti-stretch mark cream) is an excellent skin emollient. It is made by grinding roasted cacao beans and separating the vegetable fat from the product we know as chocolate.

ANTI-STRETCH MARK CREAM

An excellent cream to use during pregnancy.

10 g beeswax (grated)
10 g cocoa butter
50 ml extra virgin olive oil
75 ml grapeseed oil
35 ml orange flower water
4 drops of neroli
4 drops of lavender

98

Method:

Melt the beeswax and cocoa butter with the oils and proceed exactly as in the previous recipe.

ANTISEPTIC OINTMENT

This is a marvellous healing ointment for cuts, grazes, insect bites and stings, athlete's foot, ringworm, cold sores and chilblains. It will keep for at least 6 months due to the high concentration of essential oils.

15 g yellow beeswax (grated)
60 ml grapeseed oil
10 drops tea tree
10 drops eucalyptus
15 drops lavender

Method:
Heat the beeswax and oil in a double enamel boiler or in a heatproof basin over a pan of simmering water. Stir well, then remove from the heat. As soon as the mixture begins to thicken, stir in the essential oils then divide into little sterilized pots, cover tightly and label.

Alternative Recipe:
You could 'doctor' an unperfumed shop-bought cream with the same essential oils. Add 20 drops in all to 30 g of cream, stir in with the handle of a teaspoon. For a cooling foot balm (which also heals athlete's foot), add up to 6 drops of peppermint essence to the blend in place of the 10 drops of eucalyptus.

HAY-FEVER BALM

Having emphasized the importance of using natural oils and waxes for ointments and skin creams, no doubt you will be surprised to discover that vaseline is the main ingredient in this recipe. The vaseline acts merely as a carrier for the essential oils, which can thus evaporate and enter the nasal cavities without being absorbed itself by the skin. Apply a very small amount to the nostrils and/or rub a little into the chest at night. The balm can also be used as a symptomatic treatment for other respiratory ailments such as catarrh, 'flu and sinusitis.

1 dessertspoonful of vaseline
5 drops of eucalyptus
5 drops of pine

Method:
Melt the vaseline in a small bowl placed over a saucepan of simmering water. Remove from the heat and stir in the essential oils. Pour the mixture into a little glass pot, cover tightly and label.

HEALING LIP SALVE

This should be applied generously to dry, sore or cracked lips. The tiny quantity of peppermint oil used in this recipe will give the salve a faint minty flavour.
1 teaspoonful of grated yellow beeswax
3 teaspoonsful of almond oil
1 or 2 drops of peppermint

Method:
Melt the beeswax and oil in a small bowl placed over a saucepan of simmering water. Remove from the heat and stir in the peppermint oil. Pour into a little glass pot, cover tightly and label.

Skin Tonics

Cider vinegar is included in all the recipes for skin tonics (and also scalp treatments) because it helps to restore the skin's natural acid/alkali balance. Apply to the skin after washing or cleansing.

First choose an appropriate base for your skin type:

All skin types — distilled water.

Dry to normal skin — orange flower water or a 50/50 mixture of orange flower water and distilled water.

Normal to oily skin — rosewater or a 50/50 mixture of rosewater and distilled water.

Oily skin and acne — witch hazel or a 50/50 mixture of witch hazel and distilled water.

Method:
Funnel 300 ml of your chosen base into a dark glass bottle, then add 1 or 2 teaspoonsful of cider vinegar. Add 2 or 3 drops of an appropriate essential oil for your skin type (see page 91). Shake well each time before use.

AFTERSHAVE

Commercial products often contain alcohol and synthetic fragrances which can irritate sensitive skin. The above skin tonic blend makes an excellent gently antiseptic, yet pleasantly aromatic aftershave.

Hair Tonics

These are massaged into the scalp several times a week. If used regularly, they will improve the condition of your hair and scalp. There is no need to wet your hair first. Choose an appropriate base for your hair and scalp condition, e.g. orange flower water for dry hair, witch hazel for oily hair (see skin tonic bases above) and up to 15 drops of essential oil.

FOR DANDRUFF

If your hair is very dry, you may prefer to use the same essential oils in the deep conditioning treatment suggested on page 97.

300 ml distilled water or an appropriate floral water.
3 teaspoonsful of cider vinegar
6 drops of cedarwood
6 drops of lavender
3 drops of camomile

Method:
Funnel the water into a dark glass bottle, add the cider vinegar and the essential oils. Shake well each time before use.

Alternative Essences:
Juniper, rosemary, tea tree.

FOR STIMULATING HEALTHY HAIR GROWTH

300 ml distilled water or a floral water of your choice
3 teaspoonsful of cider vinegar
7 drops of rosemary
5 drops of sandalwood

Method:
Mix the water and oils together as in the previous recipe.

Alternative Essence:
Patchouli.

Preparations for the Mouth

Unlike most synthetic mouthwashes and breath fresheners, those containing essential oils act to retard the proliferation of bacteria. Combined with scrupulous dental hygiene, the following recipe is a healing, antiseptic mixture which will strengthen the gums, help to heal mouth ulcers and prevent the onset of gingivitis. The base ingredient, tincture of myrrh, is available from herbalists.

MOUTHWASH

30 ml tincture of myrrh
10 drops of peppermint

Method:
Mix the ingredients together and shake well.

How to use:
Rinse the mouth with 6—8 drops in a small teacupful of warm water two or three times a day.

Alternative Essences:
Fennel, geranium, tea tree.

Face Packs

Most skins (except the very sensitive) will benefit from a weekly face pack. These are designed to deep cleanse, tighten and brighten, moisturize and generally tone the complexion. One of the most beneficial substances to use as a face pack is yoghurt (live natural yoghurt, full-fat if possible) — beneficial, that is, if you are not allergic to dairy products. Fresh live yoghurt, without additives, can help all skin types, particularly excessively dry or oily skin. The lactic acid of yoghurt (due to its fermentation) is similar to that of the skin acid mantle, and appears to exert a balancing action on the secretion of skin fluids.

Another wonderful healing and moisturizing agent is raw honey, that is to say, honey that has not been subjected to pasturization. It draws moisture from the air and imparts a soft dewy glow to the complexion. Honey is suitable for all skin types — from the driest to the oiliest.

Oily, sallow or fatigued skin will benefit enormously from a face pack containing Brewer's yeast powder (available from health shops). Brewer's yeast cleanses, nourishes, tightens and tones the skin. Very oily or acneous skin may need the deep cleansing powers of Fuller's Earth, a powdered clay with wonderful skin healing properties. The same quantity of Fuller's Earth can be used to replace Brewer's yeast in the face pack suggested for oily skin and acne.

Oatmeal or ground almonds can be used as a binding agent for face packs. Oatmeal is cleansing, softening and nourishing for all skin types. Ground almonds smooth and soften drier skin.

When mixing face packs, include an essential oil suitable for your skin condition (see page 91). Otherwise, use lavender, which is a good for all skins.

FOR 'NORMAL', COMBINATION AND AGEING COMPLEXIONS

3 teaspoonsful of live, full-fat natural yoghurt
1 teaspoonful of honey
1 teaspoonful of cold-pressed vegetable oil
1 drop of essential oil
1 to 2 teaspoonsful of oatmeal to bind

Method:
Mix the essential oil into the base oil and stir in the other ingredients to form a paste. Apply a thin layer to face and neck, but keep well away from the eye area. Leave on for 10—15 minutes; rinse off with cool water.

FOR DRY SKIN

3 teaspoonsful of live, full-fat natural yoghurt
1 teaspoonful of honey
1 teaspoonful of cold-pressed vegetable oil
1 drop of essential oil
1 or 2 teaspoonsful of ground almonds

Method:
Mix and apply to the skin as in the previous recipe.

FOR OILY SKIN AND ACNE

2 teaspoonsful of live, full-fat natural yoghurt
1½ teaspoonsful of Brewer's yeast powder
½ teaspoonful of jojoba oil
1 or 2 teaspoonsful of warm water (more if necessary)
1 drop of essential oil

Method:

Mix together the jojoba and essential oil, then add the other ingredients to form a smooth paste. Oily or congested skin does not readily absorb substances unless warm and moist. Therefore it is important to apply the face pack after a bath or facial sauna. Leave on for 15 to 20 minutes and rinse off with cool water.

MOISTURIZING FACE PACK FOR ALL SKINS

2 teaspoonsful of honey
1 drop of essential oil

Method:

Stir the essential oil into the honey and apply to face and neck. Leave on for 15 to 20 minutes, preferably whilst relaxing in a warm, steamy bath. Rinse off with cool water — and admire the youthful, dewy glow!

7 · Psychic Scents

Time and time again it has been observed that we are instinctively drawn to the essential oil that is right for our needs at the time and, as our emotional state alters, so might our aroma preference. In fact, quite recently I was reminded of this phenomenon when I met a young woman at an aromatherapy conference. Interestingly, she has a love/hate relationship with camomile. More often than not, she dislikes the aroma intensely, yet during her pre-menstrual phase she craves it as much as some women long for chocolate at this time. If you look up the properties of camomile in Chapter 3, you will see that it is indeed a helpful oil for PMS and, in fact, for most other problems associated with menstruation. As for chocolate, its comforting effect may be partly due to vanilla, which is used to enhance the flavour. Vanilla is also an intriguing aroma, but more about that later.

Then there is a teenage girl of my acquaintance who is emotionally addicted to valerian essence, an unpleasant aroma beloved by cats. Sadly, she suffers from anorexia nervosa. I suspect that her obsession with the aroma is a reflection of her emotional state — that of self-torture and self-disgust. Interestingly, valerian is known to be a powerful sedative. In the past, it was used to treat nervous unrest, insomnia, St Vitus's dance, neuralgic pain and all manner of complaints generally regarded as nervous in origin. In fact, valerian is still regarded by herbalists as one of the most useful medicines for such complaints.

But what about blends of essential oils? Usually I dislike both vetiver and clary sage as individual entities, yet during a distressing episode in my life, I developed a need for a blend of these two oils. The aroma of clary and vetiver in harmony is reminiscent of the wonderful earthy scent of damp woodland, in particular, of the enchanting wood I once walked through as a child on holiday in Cornwall. Even now as I write of this aroma, the image of a mossy oak tree with spreading gnarled roots embraces my mind, offering strength and comfort, rather like a kindly weather-beaten father to my 'inner child'.

Could a disagreeable essence, then, hold the key to a hidden aspect of the psyche, an aspect requiring expression? If so, in order that we may open the door to this secret garden, we must discover the essence (or essences) with the power to turn the key in the lock, perhaps by highlighting or diminishing certain characteristics of the disliked aroma. In so doing, we create something new — an aroma that is in harmony with the soul.

So, by blending different essential oils, we not only improve the aroma of a single essence, we also influence the aroma-therapeutic effect of the end product, which of course is the essence of successful blending. There is always an aromatic blend to suit the ever changing pattern of the 'mindbody'.

Before we look at the fascinating art of blending mood-enhancing perfumes, let us consider how we might get to know the individual oils on an intuitive level.

Attunement

You may at first plump for oils that smell pretty, sensuous, spicy, refreshing or in some way familiar. That's fine if you simply wish to make an attractive perfume. However, aromatherapy proper is about exploring the deeper aspects of an aroma: the way it speaks to you personally. So, instead of taking a whiff directly from the bottle, then moving swiftly to the next, regard the art of smelling essences as a form of meditation. Put one drop of an interesting oil into the palm of your hand. Then inhale slowly and deeply, allowing yourself to fully experience its effect. Stay with the essence for at least five minutes. What does the aroma make you think of? Is it a feeling, memory or image you would like to have more often?

In fact, it may even be healing to explore the negative impressions an aroma may evoke and to write about your feelings in depth. The purpose of writing is to externalize or make more concrete that which hitherto has had the advantage of being able to work in the dark of the unconscious. It is by viewing a disturbing feeling, memory or image in the sunlight of conscious awareness that it becomes less threatening, perhaps totally disempowered. However, should an aroma association be overwhelming (a rare occurrence, though possible), perhaps stemming from some half-forgotten childhood trauma, it would be advisable to seek the aid of an accredited counsellor or therapist who will help you to work through the feelings, thus enabling you to release them into the present. A progressive therapist may even encourage you to work with the essential oil in therapy sessions.

At risk of influencing or spoiling your first impression of cypress essence, I put forward my own feelings about the oil. It has an odour that one would not immediately associate with perfume as it is somewhat medicinal-smelling, yet I find its cooling pine-like scent most intriguing. It engenders what I can only describe as an expansive sensation. As well as clearing my head, it evokes a rather solemn image of a lone cypress tree on the horizon of a vast empty plain, standing tall and silent, its dark green branches reaching up to a wide grey sky — almost sad, yet hauntingly tranquil. It is an essence which brings comfort and stillness when I am in need of quietude. What does the aroma of cypress do for you?

The Making of Perfumes

At one time all perfumes were made using essential oils. Today, alas, natural essences hardly get a look in. Indeed, you would be surprised if you knew exactly what went into some of the big-name perfumes. A beautiful bottle may contain a veritable cocktail of aroma chemicals. Yet to the highly trained nose of a top perfumier, nothing could be more crude than the use of unmodified essential oils. True, essential oils do not smell like the synthetic formulae to which many have become accustomed, but once weaned onto natural products and drawn into the healing auras of plant essences, you will never again fall for the charms of the latest 'Henry', or crave a fix of 'Venom', nor even be allured by an 'Evening in Paradise'!

Commercial perfumes are usually suspended in ethyl alcohol, but this is not generally available in Britain without a perfumier's licence, although in some countries it is readily available from pharmacies. However, alcohol is very drying to the skin. For this reason, aromatherapists tend to favour oil or beeswax-based perfumes which also have the advantage of lingering on the skin for much longer. Essential oils can also be partially suspended in distilled water or floral water to form very good aromatic waters or colognes.

While some commercial perfumes may be composed of hundreds of compounds, an aromatherapeutic perfume will rarely contain more than seven essences, perhaps as few as two or three. The reason is simple: add one essence too many and suddenly the aroma becomes irretrievably 'murky'. Similarly, if you try to blend more than a handful of pigments from a paintbox, the result is always a muddy brown no matter how bright the individual colours.

As you may know, the same perfume will smell different on different people, especially those of the opposite sex. This is because the aromatic molecules interact with our own body chemistry, changing from one moment to the next. As the essences evaporate, different nuances of the fragrance become apparent; the aroma shape-changes on the skin, plays hide-and-seek with the senses until finally it disappears into the ether, leaving nothing but the memory of its sweet embrace.

A Fragrant Symphony

In simple terms, a 'well-balanced' perfume is composed of top notes, middle notes and base notes, just like music. The top notes of a perfume are highly volatile — they do not last very long. These are essences such as bergamot, lemon and coriander. They form the scent's first impression, giving brightness and clarity to the blend, much as a flute adds high-pitched purity to an orchestra. The middle or 'heart' notes last a little longer;

109

they impart warmth and fullness to the perfume. Rose otto, geranium and ylang ylang are some of the most popular middle notes. Then there are the heavier-smelling, deeply resonating base notes which have a profound influence on the blend as a whole: patchouli, vetiver and sandalwood. They are very long-lasting and at the same time, they 'fix' other essences. This means they slow down the volatility rate of the top and middle notes, thus improving on the 'staying power' of the perfume.

Some essential oils are good 'bridges' — they connect individual components and allow them to blend. Thus the perfume begins to resonate as a harmonious whole, much as the vibrations of individual instruments in an orchestra combine to create a symphony.

A single essential oil may vibrate mainly from the base, yet nuances of the aroma may also reach up to the middle pitch, thus the essence can be used to connect the base notes of a blend with the heart. Cedarwood and frankincense are such bridges. Another bridging essence may resonate mainly from the top, yet also connect with the middle (bergamot, basil). Similarly, a heart note may also span the upper sphere (geranium, clary sage), or reach down towards the base (ylang ylang, cypress). However, the bridging note supreme must surely be rose otto, for although resonating mainly from the heart, it also embraces both head and base. For this reason it makes a wonderful perfume all by itself — or perhaps I am more than a little biased by my own aroma preference!

Good bridging notes are those which resonate from more than one level. The most commonly used bridges include bergamot, cedarwood, clary sage, frankincense, geranium, lavender, neroli, rose otto, sandalwood and ylang ylang.

To take an example, should your blend smell too garish, the top note being far removed from the heart note, the blend can be brought into harmony by adding an essential oil that vibrates from the middle towards the upper sphere — rose otto or clary sage would be a good choice. If, on the other hand, the base note has become too pronounced, having no connection with the heart, you would need to 'lift' the aroma by adding an essence that resonates from middle to base: rose otto or ylang

ylang, for instance. Should the base note still be predominant, continue to build the perfume by adding a few drops of an essence that resonates from middle to top: lavender, clary sage or geranium.

Of course, you may decide to use all top notes in a blend; a traditional *eau de cologne* mixture perhaps, composed mainly of citrus oils. Or a blend composed entirely of middle notes, or of base notes — or whatever permutation you can think of. However, should you opt for all top notes, do not expect the fragrance to be anything more than a brief encounter.

If you are beginning to feel perplexed about creative blending, you can choose to ignore all this about perfume notes if you wish — many aromatherapists do. After all, the rules were devised by perfumiers rather than therapists. Just like a naïve painter, untrained singer or musician, you too can create more than adequate compositions coloured by your own unique essence. Simply be guided by your faithful nose, keep practising and before long you will compose that masterpicce!

However, if you are determined to blend according to rule, the following list may help. It categorizes all the essential oils mentioned in Chapter 3 (and a few others) according to their perfume notes. The information given is also relevant to the blending of massage oils and room perfumes. Incidentally, for those who would delight in the antiseptic aroma of tea tree (not usually an essence employed in perfumery) the oil is categorized as a top note — whatever turns you on, as they say!

TOP NOTES

Angelica	Fennel	Mandarin
Basil	Grapefruit	Orange
Bergamot	Lavender	Peppermint
Cardomom	Lemon	Petitgrain
Coriander	Lemongrass	Tea tree
Eucalyptus	Lime	

TOP TO MIDDLE

Angelica
Basil
Bergamot
Cardomom

Fennel
Geranium
Lavender
Lemongrass

Neroli
Petitgrain
Tagetes

MIDDLE TO TOP

Black Pepper
Camomile
Clary Sage
Clove (*as a room perfume*)

Geranium
Juniper
Lavender
Neroli

Palma Rosa
Pine Needle
Rose Otto

MIDDLE NOTES

Black Pepper
Cinnamon Bark
  (*as a room perfume*)
Clary Sage
Clove
  (*as a room perfume*)

Geranium
Ginger
Juniper
Lavender
Marjoram
Neroli

Pine Needle
Palma Rosa
Rose Otto
Rosemary
Vanilla
Ylang Ylang

MIDDLE TO BASE

Cypress
Myrrh

Rose Otto
Vanilla

Ylang Ylang

BASE TO MIDDLE

Cedarwood
Frankincense

Myrrh
Sandalwood

BASE NOTES

Cedarwood
Frankincense

Patchouli
Sandalwood

Vetiver

Developing a Theme

Broadly speaking, there are four families of scent — floral, chypre, green and oriental — though most will have overtones of another as well. Each family has its own fascination and will appeal to a particular personality or a particular mood. Indeed, so workable are these themes that I have chosen to use them as a framework for the open-ended recipe section of this chapter.

Floral: A simple blend created to emanate a single floral note such as rose or neroli, or a harmonious bouquet without any particular flower predominating — essentially feminine.

Chypre: Reminiscent of dark green woods after rain. The blend may be developed from a base of vetiver and clary sage, with perhaps a bridge of cypress, sandalwood or cedarwood and a mysterious veil of frankincense. A tinge of citrus or of rose creates a shaft of sunlight through the trees. A long-lasting, sensuous perfume which appeals to both men and women.

Green: Sharp and clear, reminiscent of the great outdoors. The blend may be developed from a base of clary sage and an evergreen essence such as cedarwood, pine, juniper or cypress, perhaps made greener by a tinge of an herbaceous essence such as basil or rosemary and heightened with an exhilarating breeze of lime. A sporty, 'get-up-and-go' fragrance, essentially androgynous.

Oriental: A sultry, full-bodied blend composed of deeply resonating essences such as patchouli and sandalwood, exotic florals and spices, and the oils of luscious fruits. A tenacious, overtly seductive scent for the bold at heart!

Prelude

113

Before going ahead and mixing a quantity of perfume as directed in the recipe section, you will need to find out whether or not the blend is compatible with your personality or present mood. For there is nothing more disappointing than to discover that an enchanting-sounding blend is totally out of synch with your own magical expectations, especially if you are left with a full bottle of the offending brew. No doubt you will also wish to experiment with blends of your own devising. Here, then, are a few economical methods for smell-testing your aromatic concoctions.

1. Put a drop or two of each essential oil on a *damp* cotton bud, a smelling stick (available from essential oil suppliers) or a piece of blotting paper. Before smelling, waft the sample around for a moment to encourage vaporization of the essences. If you dislike the effect, you have wasted only a small amount of essential oil.
2. A more accurate guide would be to mix the sample combination of oils (up to 6 drops in all) in a teaspoonful of light coconut oil or jojoba and apply to the inside of your wrist before smelling. The oils will then have the chance to interact with your skin chemistry. If you like the effect, mix to perfume strength.
3. For the testing of aromatic waters and room perfumes, add up to 6 drops of essential oil to 2 teaspoonsful of warm water and mix well. If you dislike the effect, sprinkle the mixture over the area where the dog or cat usually sleeps! (N.B. Some oils, patchouli, for example, may stain cotton fabric; however, any stain should only be temporary as the oil eventually evaporates.)

Incidentally, you may have to limit yourself to testing no more than six blends or six different essences at a time. The nose becomes fatigued after that and therefore less discerning.

Most important:
You will need a notebook in which to accurately record your successful formulas (and perhaps also your failures). It is so easy to forget.

CAUTION:
The quantity of essential oil in perfume blends is quite high. So, if you have very sensitive skin or know you have an allergy to

114

perfume, you may have to forego the delights of wearing even a natural skin perfume. However, you could perfume cotton outer garments with an aromatic water or enjoy room perfumes instead.

Odour Intensity Guide

The following essential oils have very powerful aromas and will dominate your blends unless used in small quantities. The amount suggested for each essence is for 10 ml of jojoba or light coconut oil for perfume making, 25 ml of vegetable oil for massage blends and 100 ml of water for room perfumes and colognes. If the aroma appears to be too weak, add an extra drop, shake well, then sniff. Add another drop if necessary — more if you dare!

Basil: 1 or 2 drops
Black Pepper: 1 or 2 drops
Cardomom: 1 drop
Camomile: 1 or 2 drops
Cinnamon Bark (room perfume only): 2 or 3 drops
Clove (room perfume only): 2 or 3 drops
Eucalyptus: 1 drop
Fennel: 1 to 3 drops
Frankincense: 1 to 3 drops
Ginger: 1 or 2 drops
Lemongrass: 1 or 2 drops
Myrrh: 1 or 2 drops
Neroli: 2 to 4 drops
Peppermint: 1 or 2 drops
Rose Otto: 1 to 3 drops
Tagetes: 1 drop

Oil-Based Perfumes

Although the following open-ended recipes are based on the four families of scent (floral, chypre, green and oriental), this still leaves plenty of scope for you to develop your own ideas. Each formula is built in two or three stages, so if you discover you love the first part and wish to go no further, simply make up to perfume strength by adjusting the quantity of essential oil accordingly.

Basic Procedure:

Fill a 10 ml dark glass bottle almost to the top with light coconut oil or jojoba. Build your perfume slowly drop by drop, shaking the bottle after each addition and smelling as you go. You will need between 15 and 20 drops altogether. Begin with the base note (if included), then develop the heart of the perfume and finally the top note.

Once mixed, your perfume needs to be left for one or two weeks to mature. Keep it in a cool dark place, but remember to shake the bottle once a day to facilitate the process. At the end of the maturation period, the blend will have lost its 'raw' overtone and will smell altogether more rounded. But if it seems to be too strong, dilute it with a little more jojoba or light coconut oil.

Floral Perfumes

For a light bouquet, begin with a base mixture of 3 drops of ylang ylang and 5 drops of geranium. Develop the theme by adding up to 10 drops in all of 2 or 3 of the following essences: lavender, clary sage, petitgrain, neroli (no more than 2 drops), bergamot, mandarin or grapefruit.

For a long-lasting sensuous bouquet, begin with a base of 6 drops of patchouli, cedarwood or sandalwood (or a combination of any two), then develop the heart by adding up to 8 drops in all of 2 or 3 of the following essences: clary sage, geranium, lavender, rose otto (no more than 2 drops) or ylang ylang. For the top note, add up to 5 drops of bergamot, mandarin or orange.

SUGGESTED BLENDS

(Measurements given in drops.)

1. Ylang-ylang 3, geranium 5, lavender 3, clary sage 3, bergamot 4.
2. Cedarwood 6, ylang ylang 6, rose otto 2, grapefruit 5.
3. Patchouli 6, cedarwood 3, neroli 3, geranium 3, clary sage 3.

Chypre Perfumes

To create the dark green atmosphere of a damp mossy wood, begin with 5 drops of vetiver or patchouli and 5 drops of clary sage. To bridge these 2 essences, you could add 3 drops of cedarwood, sandalwood or cypress. To further develop an aura of mystery, add 1 or 2 drops of frankincense. Should you wish to bring in some dappled sunlight to dance on the woodland carpet, add up to 5 drops in all of 1 or 2 of the following essences: bergamot, grapefruit, lime, mandarin, neroli (1 or 2 drops), petitgrain, rose otto (1 or 2 drops).

SUGGESTED BLENDS

1. Vetiver 6, clary sage 6, cypress 3, grapefruit 3, petitgrain 2.
2. Patchouli 5, clary sage 5, sandalwood 6, rose otto 2.
3. Vetiver 6, clary sage 3, cedarwood 3, frankincense 2, bergamot 5.

Green Perfumes

To create a feeling of fresh air and high places, begin with a base mixture of 5 drops of clary sage and up to 7 drops in all of 1 or 2 of the following evergreen essences: cedarwood, cypress, juniper or pine. Develop the theme by adding 1 drop of basil or rosemary and/or 2 drops of lavender. For an exhilarating effect, you might dare to add a single drop of peppermint. Complete the picture by adding up to 6 drops in all of any of the following essences: grapefruit, lemon, lime (no more than 3 drops), neroli (1 or 2 drops), petitgrain. For a warm tinge, include a few drops of bergamot.

SUGGESTED BLENDS

1. Cypress 5, clary sage 5, lavender 4, neroli 2, lemon 3.
2. Cedarwood 3, juniper 3, clary sage 5, basil 1, bergamot 6.
3. Juniper 6, clary sage 6, lavender 3, rosemary 1, peppermint 1, lime 3
4. Cedarwood 5, pine 5, clary sage 5, lime 3, lemon 2.

Oriental Perfumes

Definitely not for the faint-hearted! Begin with a deeply resonating base composed of 5 drops of patchouli and 5 drops of cedarwood. Or you might prefer a base mixture of one or more of the following essences: frankincense, myrrh, sandalwood or vetiver. For a seductive warm glow, add up to 6 drops in all of 2 or more of the following heart notes: ginger (1 or 2 drops), marjoram, rose otto (up to 3 drops), ylang ylang. For the top note of this luscious brew, add up to 5 drops in all of one or two of the following essences: bergamot, cardomom (no more than 1 drop), coriander, grapefruit, lavender, lemon, lime, mandarin, neroli, orange.

SUGGESTED BLENDS

1. Patchouli 5, ylang ylang 5, frankincense 3, rose otto 3, coriander 4.
2. Sandalwood 6, ylang ylang 6, ginger 1, marjoram 3, bergamot 4.
3. Cedarwood 4, frankincense 5, myrrh 4, cardomom 1, lavender 3, lime 3.

Solid Perfumes

These are very simple to make, and are rather like the ointment recipe in the previous chapter:

SOLID PERFUME

1 level teaspoonful of grated beeswax
2 teaspoonsful (10 ml) of jojoba or light coconut oil.
25–30 drops of essential oil.

Method:
Blend the essential oils with the jojoba or coconut oil as in
the previous recipes. Melt the beeswax in a small heatproof
bowl placed over a milk saucepan of simmering water.
Remove from the heat and stir in the perfume blend. Pour
into a little sterilized glass pot, cover tightly and label.

The honey-scented beeswax adds its own subtle fragrance to the
blend. You can incorporate any of the aforementioned formulas
into the beeswax base, adjusting the quantity of essential oil
accordingly. Or you might like to develop a theme of your own.

Aromatic Waters

Although essential oils are only partially soluble in water, they
can be made into most acceptable aromatic waters or colognes –
– especially if poured through a coffee filter paper to clarify the
mixture. This also reduces, to a degree, any separation of
essential oil and water. Again, you can develop a fragrance based
on one of the four families of scent or devise your own. If you
love the warm aroma of vanilla, you could incorporate real
vanilla extract to water-based blends (see page 138). Or you
may prefer one of the *eau de cologne* formulas as suggested below.
These can be used in the same way as commercial products —
splashed on after a bath or shower, brushed through the hair
or sprinkled over cotton garments.

Basic Procedure:
Pour into a dark glass bottle 100 ml in all of distilled water,
orange flower water or rosewater, or a 50/50 mixture of any
two. Then build the fragrance gradually, adding a few drops of
essential oil, shaking the mixture well and smelling as you go.

As with oil-based perfumes, the mixture will improve if it is allowed to ripen for 1 or 2 weeks before use. Keep in a cool dark place, but remember to shake well each day as you pass by. When ready, pour through a coffee filter paper, rebottle and label.

SUGGESTED *EAU DE COLOGNE* BLENDS

Classic:
   40 drops bergamot
   10 drops petitgrain
   10 drops orange
   25 drops lemon
   10 drops lavender
    5 drops rosemary

Luxury:
   15 drops neroli
    4 drops rose otto
   15 drops grapefruit
   10 drops lemon
   30 drops bergamot
   14 drops mandarin
   10 drops orange

Spicy:
   20 drops bergamot
   20 drops orange
   10 drops lavender
   10 drops coriander
   10 drops frankincense
   10 drops petitgrain
    5 drops lime

8 · Ambience in the Making

Of all the methods of perfuming rooms, there is nothing quite like the magic of a purpose-designed essential oil vaporizer, or 'burner' as they are often called. They are beautiful to look at — usually earthenware (sometimes glass, porcelain or marble), with petal-shaped openings cut out of the sides to afford a free flow of air for the nightlight candle which is placed inside. A small detachable reservoir fits over the nightlight and is filled with a previously prepared aromatic water. Alternatively, the reservoir is filled with plain water and a few drops of essential oil floated on the surface. This is gently heated by the flame. As the aromatic water evaporates, the room becomes permeated with fragrance. If burned in a dimly lit or darkened room, floral patterns dance on the wall like shadow puppets. The elements of earth (the clay), fire (the flame), water and air (the aromatic vapour) combine, creating an ambience of enchantment.

There is one drawback, however: if you forget to refill the reservoir after the water has evaporated (which can be quite soon with some vaporizers) you may be left with a sticky, blackened residue of burnt oil. This can be difficult to remove, unless you use an alcohol-based substance such as surgical spirit. Nevertheless, to my mind this is a small price to pay for an otherwise delightful effect.

An electric fragrancer is the high-tech alternative. Here a few drops of undiluted essential oil is dropped on to a ceramic or filter surface which is kept at a constant warm temperature. There is just enough heat to release the aromatic vapour without risk of burning. These gadgets are particularly suitable for the workplace and certainly much safer for children's bedrooms.

The most recent innovation is the stream diffuser. A cold-air pump blows minuscule droplets of neat essential oil into the atmosphere. The advantage of this method is that the essential oil is not subjected to heat which, if too fierce, can radically alter its chemical structure.

However, a well-designed essential oil burner (or electric vaporizer) should not cause the oils to overheat. But there are still some very poorly designed burners on the market, often with the nightlight too close to the reservoir, which means the aromatic water can actually reach boiling point! Moreover, you may be sold an inadequately ventilated burner which, though aesthetically pleasing, causes the nightlight to suffocate after a short while. In fact, I have two such useless pieces of equipment (bought several years ago), one of which is afflicted with both problems! So it is important to obtain vaporizing equipment from a reputable supplier (see addresses in the Appendix). A few outlets, particularly craft shops, often display a sample burner in full use, which of course is the most reliable guide to its effectiveness.

Blending for the Vapourizer

If you opt for an electric vaporizer or diffuser, the essential oils must be used neat. As few as 3 or 4 drops of essential oil are usually enough to perfume a room up to 3 metres square. For a much larger space, you may need up to 15 drops. You may find it easier to blend several undiluted essential oils together in a single bottle and to put a few drops of the blend on the ceramic plate or filter surface. However, before going ahead and blending the oils, it is important to ensure that the effect will be pleasing, otherwise you may have wasted a large amount of essential oil. Therefore, it would be wise to aroma test your blends as suggested for perfume making (see page 118).

When making blends for the nightlight vaporizer, you will need to mix 15—20 drops of essential oil to a 100—125 ml bottle of water. Then fill the oil burner reservoir with some of the blend. But do remember to shake the bottle each time before use. For special occasions, you could mix the essential oils with rosewater or orange flower water, which is especially lovely with floral or citrus essences.

Aromas for the Workplace

As we have already seen, the effect of aroma is highly subjective. For this reason, it can be something of a juggling act to create an environmental aroma to please everyone.

So, unless you are fortunate enough to have an office or workspace to yourself, do seek your colleagues' approval before subjecting them to mood-enhancing fragrance, as it might be construed as rather 'Big Brotherish' otherwise! Having gained their enthusiasm, it is also important to check that the aroma is, at the very least, acceptable to everyone. It may be too much to expect all of your colleagues to adore the fragrance, but for obvious reasons it is important to ensure that no one actively dislikes it.

Generally speaking, the most popular environmental fragrances for the workplace are those from either the green or citrus families — essences such as pine, cypress, juniper, lemon, orange, lime, bergamot or grapefruit. They can be used singly or in blends. Although it cannot be guaranteed that everyone will be happy with these aromas, in my experience, very few would object. The green scents conjure up feelings of the great outdoors, most welcome to the average indoor worker. The citrus essences, especially orange, bergamot and mandarin, add an uplifting, jolly note to blends. Moreover, many essential oils are excellent fumigants, helping to prevent the spread of bacteria, and even viruses, in stuffy workplaces — most helpful during the winter months when almost everyone seems to have a cold. In fact, eucalyptus and tea tree oils are the most efficacious in this respect. They can be blended with lemon and/or lavender to improve the aroma.

SUGGESTED BLENDS

1. Cypress, petitgrain, bergamot.
2. Pine, eucalyptus, lemon.
3. Lavender, rosemary, grapefruit.

Recipes

The quantity of oil used in the following recipes will vary, depending on the size of the workspace (refer back to *Blending for the Vapourizer*, page 126). It is advisable to use an electric vaporizer for the workplace rather than a nightlight burner, which could represent a fire hazard.

For mental work of any nature, you may find basil, rosemary or peppermint helpful. These essences have traditionally been credited with 'cephalic' properties, i.e. they stimulate clarity of thought. However, I would also include eucalyptus, pine and juniper in this category. When inhaled, these essences (especially peppermint) are cooling to the respiratory tract. They also help to loosen sinus catarrh, thus inducing a clear-headed sensation. Incidentally, mint-flavoured sweets are very popular with students, especially during examinations. This is an example of an instinctive ability to know which aroma (or flavour) we need at any given time. A healthier alternative would be to sprinkle a few drops of peppermint on a handkerchief and inhale as required — though admittedly, this is not quite as enjoyable as sucking mints!

Other uplifting, head-clearing essences include lemon, bergamot, grapefruit and coriander. You may also find an *eau de cologne* formula conducive to mental work (see the recipes on page 124).

SUGGESTED BLENDS

1. Basil, bergamot, coriander.
2. Juniper, lemon.
3. Eucalyptus, grapefruit, bergamot.

Aromas for your Home

As long as other members of the family do not object, the essential oil blends you use in the home can be as adventurous as you like. You could base your creations on any of the aroma families suggested in the previous chapter — floral, chypre, green and oriental — or you could use simple blends of two or three essences to suit the room, the season or the occasion.

If you do not own an essential oil vaporizer or an electric diffuser, there are other methods of perfuming rooms, not only for aesthetic purposes, but also to help prevent the spread of infection during epidemics (see page 80).

You could also vaporize essential oils in the molten wax of a burning candle — a method which I learned from the proprietor of a shop specializing in candles! However, it is important to obtain a very fat candle which will produce a good-sized pool of wax around the wick, thus enabling the oil to vaporize slowly.

The method is as follows: first light the candle. Wait for the wax to melt, then blow it out and immediately add a few drops of essential oil around the wick before re-lighting. Essential oil is highly flammable, so if you attempt to add this whilst the candle is still burning, it will flare up, leaving in its wake a puff of black smoke. It is also important to keep the wick trimmed very short, otherwise the flame will be too big and the aromatic vapour relatively short-lived.

One of my own favourite methods of perfuming rooms during the winter months is to drape over radiators bunches of essential oil-impregnated pine cones which have been tied together with cotton thread. As they gradually open from the warmth of the radiator, gentle fragrance is diffused into the room.

The cones need to be soaked for at least an hour, preferably overnight, in 125 ml of water with up to 25 drops of essential oil. To keep the cones redolent with fragrance, you will need to soak them once a week. Any left-over aromatic soak-water can be poured through a coffee filter paper (to remove any debris) and used in the pottery burner.

Bunches of fragrant cones can also be hung in the wardrobe as a moth repellent. Any of the following essences are recommended for this purpose: cedarwood, citronella, lavender, lemongrass, patchouli or sandalwood. Alternatively, fill a little dish with woodshavings, then sprinkle with about 20 drops of essential oil.

125

You can also put scented handkerchiefs in the linen cupboard and in drawers to keep everything fresh and sweet-smelling. Lavender is an old-time favourite, though you may enjoy other refreshing essences such as bergamot, coriander, geranium, lemon or petitgrain.

Different Rooms, Different Moods

Once you have become familiar with a number of essential oils they will begin to speak to you. Some will feel more suitable for the kitchen; others, the bedroom, bathroom, living-room, study and so on. Although of course this is a matter of personal preference, I offer my own ideas as a basic guide. It also needs to be remembered that when blended, the oils may suggest a different mood. Take ylang ylang, for example, a sweet floral essence reminiscent of a blend of almonds and jasmine. Mix it with rose otto, neroli or lavender and its feminine, sensuous qualities are enhanced. Blend the essence with larger quantities of frankincense and lemon and a rather serious, almost 'religious' aroma is created, one which would be suited to yoga practice or meditation.

Remember that if you wish to enhance, rather than alter, the personality of an individual oil, it will need to be blended with essences of a similar nature.

Incidentally, the number of drops used in room perfumes will depend on the method of vaporization (refer back to *Blending for the Vapourizer*, page 126) and the effect you wish to create. Therefore you must let your nose be your guide. In any case, unlike blending for skin perfumes, with room perfumes exact quantities are not at all crucial.

Guide:
If you wish your blends to remain in character, *choose two or three essences* from the *same enumerated group* within the same room (see below). If you wish to add contrast, choose oils from more than one group within the same room. Or why not go Bohemian and merge the kitchen with the bedroom, the living-room with the bathroom, or the study with the toilet!

THE KITCHEN

1. Bergamot, grapefruit, lemon, lime, mandarin, orange.
2. Basil, marjoram, peppermint, rosemary.
3. Black pepper, cardomom, cinnamon bark, clove, coriander, ginger.

Hint:
Groups 1 and 3 blend well together, as do groups 1 and 2.

THE UTILITY ROOM

1. Cypress, eucalyptus, juniper, pine, rosemary.
2. Bergamot, grapefruit, lemon, lime.

Hint:
Both groups blend well together.

THE BATHROOM

1. Cypress, eucalyptus, juniper, pine, rosemary.
2. Bergamot, grapefruit, lemon, lime.
3. Geranium, lavender, petitgrain.

Hint:
All 3 groups blend well together.

THE TOILET

As for the bathroom, but with the addition of tea tree in group 1. Tea tree does not blend very well with other essences (the aroma is very intense), but it may be acceptable with eucalyptus, pine, lavender or lemon.

127

THE LIVING-ROOM/SITTING-ROOM

1. Bergamot, grapefruit, lemon, lime, mandarin, orange.
2. Cypress, juniper, pine.

3. Clary sage, geranium, lavender, neroli, petitgrain.
4. *Heavy lingering aromas for relaxation:* cedarwood, frankincense, patchouli, rose otto, sandalwood, vetiver, ylang ylang.

Hint:
Groups 1, 2 and 3 and 4 blend well together. However, rose otto is the exception, it does not blend well with group 2.

THE STUDY

1. Basil, peppermint, rosemary.
2. Cypress, eucalyptus, juniper, pine.
3. Black pepper, cardomom, coriander.
4. Bergamot, grapefruit, lemon, lime.

Hint:
Groups 1 and 4 (with the exception of peppermint) blend well together. Peppermint is best used alone. Groups 2 and 4 blend well together, as do groups 3 and 4.

THE BEDROOM

1. Camomile, clary sage, lavender.
2. Neroli, rose otto, ylang ylang.
3. Frankincense, patchouli, sandalwood, vetiver.

Hint:
Group 1 is suitable for a child's bedroom, but use half the usual concentration of essential oil, e.g. 1 or 2 drops in an electric diffuser. Groups 1, 2 and 3 blend well together. However, camomile is a little more difficult. It does not blend very well with the oils in group 3, unless used in tiny amounts, e.g. 1 drop to 100 ml of water.

128

Seasonal Aromas

You may have discovered that certain essential oils have a cooling, refreshing quality and are therefore most welcome on hot summer days and sultry nights. Other oils are warming to both body and mind, and are suitable for the wintertime. So you may enjoy blending accordingly, perhaps also discovering which oils are in harmony with spring and autumn as well. As these two seasons form a bridge between winter and summer and summer and winter respectively, this should serve as a guide. Although I have suggested a number of 'seasonal bridges', the final decision is your own — spring or autumn?

Summertime: Bergamot, clary sage, cypress, eucalyptus, geranium, grapefruit, juniper, lavender, lemon, lime, peppermint, pine.

Wintertime: Black pepper, cardomom, cinnamon bark, clove, frankincense, ginger, orange, marjoram.

Seasonal Bridges: Bergamot, cedarwood, camomile, coriander, geranium, lavender, mandarin, neroli, petitgrain, rose otto, rosemary, sandalwood, ylang ylang.

Aromas to Suit the Occasion

Just to get you started, here are some of my own favourite occasions and blends to suit — a few of which are blatantly obvious!

A CHRISTMAS PARTY

SUGGESTED BLENDS

1. Equal quantities of cinnamon bark and clove with a larger quantity of orange.
2. Equal quantities of cedarwood, frankincense and myrrh. If you find this too heavy, add a few drops of bergamot, mandarin or orange to lift the fragrance.

A CHILDREN'S PARTY

SUGGESTED BLENDS

1. Equal quantities of geranium, lavender and mandarin.
2. Equal quantities of bergamot, coriander and petitgrain.
3. Equal quantities of clary sage and lavender with a larger quantity of bergamot.

DINNER *À DEUX*

SUGGESTED BLENDS

1. Equal quantities of patchouli and ylang ylang with a smaller quantity of rose otto.
2. Use rosewater instead of plain water as your base, then add some sandalwood essence and a smaller quantity of rose otto.
3. Equal quantities of clary sage and vetiver, heightened with a few drops of geranium or neroli or ylang ylang — or a little of each.

AN EASTER CELEBRATION

Vanilla is a lovely aroma to vaporize at Eastertime. You will find a recipe for homemade vanilla extract, and some suggestions for its use in the essential oil burner, on page 138. Suffice it to say here that vanilla mixes especially well with cinnamon bark and citrus essences. Alternatively, you might prefer to vaporize one of the spicy floral blends suggested below.

SUGGESTED BLENDS

1. Equal quantities of coriander, geranium and ylang ylang.
2. Equal quantities of bergamot, geranium and lavender with a touch of cinnamon bark.

MIDSUMMER'S EVE

Astrologers believe that everything on Earth has a heavenly ruler. Therefore the most appropriate essences to vaporize for a midsummer's celebration are those which are traditionally associated with the sun. These include angelica, bergamot, black pepper, cinnamon bark, clove, ginger, juniper, lemon, melissa, orange and rosemary.

SUGGESTED BLENDS

1. Equal quantities of bergamot and juniper.
2. Equal quantities of angelica and lemon.
3. A larger quantity of bergamot, made spicy with a touch of clove.

HARVEST FESTIVAL

To represent the bountiful Earth, include one of the full-bodied essences in your blends: frankincense, patchouli, rose otto, sandalwood or vetiver. Mix this with a larger quantity of one or more of the citrus essences: bergamot, grapefruit, lemon, lime, mandarin or orange.

SUGGESTED BLENDS

1. Equal quantities of bergamot, grapefruit and orange with a smaller quantity of frankincense.
2. Equal quantities of cedarwood and frankincense, a larger quantity of mandarin, and a touch of rose otto if you wish.

HALLOWE'EN

Choose dark and mysterious essences such as patchouli or vetiver, heightened with evergreen oils such as cedarwood, cypress, juniper or pine. Clary sage is a good bridge between patchouli and vetiver and the evergreens. Just for impish fun, you might like to add some valerian essence to your Hallowe'en potion — an evil-smelling oil guaranteed to swing the witch's cat into ecstasy! But I offer no clues to its blending, nor take any responsibility for suggesting it! The choice is yours, dear reader — trick or treat?

SUGGESTED BLENDS

1. Equal quantities of cedarwood, clary sage and vetiver.
2. Equal quantities of clary sage and patchouli with a smaller quantity of juniper.

YOUR NEW HOME

Vaporizing essential oils in a new home is a lovely way to make your mark on it. Move the burner or electric diffuser from room to room, not forgetting the bathroom or toilet, until the whole house is permeated with fragrance.

As a matter of interest, a friend of mine used a blend of lavender and frankincense to 'exorcise' a room in her house which always had a strange atmosphere. Even the dog would not go in there. Every day for about a month she vaporized the essential oils, using a traditional pottery burner. After a while, to everyone's surprise, the atmosphere changed and the difference was tangible. The dog, however, proved to be the most accurate barometer, for he chose to sleep in the room. So it appears that essential oils have ghost-busting properties too! In fact, frankincense, and also juniper, have been used for thousands of years for 'cleansing' atmospheres.

It is also good to embrace your new home with music. If you can play a musical instrument or sing, then play or sing to your heart's content — but not too late into the night, unless you wish to make enemies of your new neighbours! Otherwise put on a tape or record of inspiring music. This could be the Gregorian chants, 'The Messiah' — or a heavy metal piece if that is your thing. (Musical pomposity plays no part here!)

SUGGESTED BLENDS

1. Equal quantities of frankincense and lavender.
2. Equal quantities of juniper and lavender.
3. Equal quantities of frankincense and juniper.

No doubt you can think of many other occasions and essential oils to suit. However, there is one aroma and flavour that, so far, has only been mentioned in passing, a substance worthy of much more praise: vanilla.

Rhapsody in Vanilla

The vanilla pod or bean is the fruit of the exotic climbing orchid which is native to Mexico, though the plants are now grown in all tropical areas. Vanilla is not a spice, therefore it has no essential oil. Its unique flavour and aroma come not from the living plant, but from the vanillin crystals which form on the surface of the pod. But first it must undergo a complicated process of fermentation which can take up to six months to complete. The plants also have to be hand-pollinated (unless grown in their native Mexico where indigenous orchid-pollinating insects abound). Moreover, it takes three years before the first crop can be harvested; the vines continue fruiting for a further nine. Not surprisingly then, vanilla is one of the most expensive flavourings in the world, and the reason why much of what passes for vanilla is a synthetic substance derived mainly from the sulphite by-products of the paper industry! Few people have savoured the delights of the real thing.

It was the sixteenth-century Spanish explorer Cortez who introduced vanilla to Europe. He discovered it in Mexico, where the Aztecs used it to flavour their chocolate drinks. In fact, the combination of chocolate and vanilla was deemed so emotionally powerful that Aztec women were forbidden the pleasure! However, the more liberated Spanish ladies of the New World were free to explore the delights of such heavenly nectar. Many became so addicted to vanilla-flavoured chocolate that, not content to drink it several times each day, they even had it served to them in church!

Although the medicinal value of vanilla has declined over the years, it was at one time considered to be a stimulant, an aid to digestion — and a powerful aphrodisiac!

Certainly, vanilla (along with chocolate) is one of the most seductive of flavours. Very few people remain unmoved by its smooth taste and aroma. As well as being used to flavour confectionery, vanilla is also employed by the perfumier, who

133

regards it as a middle to base note. It evokes in many people feelings of warmth and security. While chocolate is known to contain a happiness substance (the amphetamine–like chemical phenylethylamine), no one has yet explained the allure of vanilla, at least not in chemical terms.

Although it is not possible to obtain a true essential oil from vanilla pods, a solvent-extracted vanilla absolute is available — at a price. However, for reasons already put forward (see Chapter 2), I would not recommend the use of absolutes in aromatherapy.

It is possible, however, to obtain real vanilla extract or 'essence' (vanilla suspended in alcohol) from a few health shops and herbal suppliers. Although you cannot use vanilla essence in oil-based perfumes or in electric diffusers, you can incorporate it into cologne blends and water-based mixtures for use in the essential oil burner. Use ½ to 1 teaspoonful (depending on the strength of the vanilla) to 100 mls of water. Vanilla can be vaporized alone or blended with up to 20 drops of any of the following essential oils: cinnamon, citrus essences, clove (a tiny amount), geranium, neroli, patchouli, petitgrain, rose otto, sandalwood and ylang ylang.

The addition of vanilla essence to aromatic waters will cause the mixture to turn cloudy, which may not matter for your own use. However, should you wish to make a vanilla blend as a gift, leave it to stand overnight. Next day, shake well, then pour through a coffee filter paper to clarify the mixture.

You may enjoy making your own vanilla extract from a vanilla pod steeped in vodka. If you have never seen a vanilla pod before, you may at first wonder how such a dry and wrinkled tendril could possibly produce anything remotely aromatic. You are about to be amazed!

VANILLA EXTRACT

1 vanilla pod
50 ml vodka

Method:
Split the vanilla pod lengthwise, then put it into a glass jar or jug and cover with vodka. Cover the jar and allow to steep for at least six weeks. Even when ready to use (in cooking and/or for making aromatic waters) leave the vanilla pod in the vodka. You will find that the mixture continues to strengthen, which means you can add a little more vodka if you wish. A particularly redolent pod will take an extra 50 ml.

VANILLA ROOM-PERFUMES

Vanilla base:
100 ml of water, ½ to 1 teaspoonful of vanilla essence.

1.   8 drops of ylang ylang, 8 drops of geranium, 1 drop of clove.
2. 10 drops of ylang ylang, 6 drops of lime.
3. 12 drops of sandalwood, 2 drops of rose otto.

Fragrant Earth

The most natural form of aromatherapy comes to us free — from the great outdoors. What better way to experience the aromas of herbs, flowers, trees and grasses than directly as nature intended. Even moist earth smells wonderful, especially during hot weather, when the first summer rains fall on the parched meadows like tears of joy. Then there is the warm, sweet scent of honeysuckle lingering on the air of a sultry summer's evening, and the cooling aromas of pine, cedar and cypress. Instinctively, we breathe more deeply in order to fully experience their aromas — and the more deeply and fully we breathe, the more relaxed and in harmony we feel. For nature in her myriad forms offers tranquillity to the frenzied and raises the spirits of the down-hearted. All that she asks in return is a little of our time and attention. Even if you live far from the countryside, the local park can be a source of healing. So try to take some time out each day simply to commune with nature — to walk on the grass, to touch the rough bark of an ancient tree, to listen to the birds, to breathe in the scents of plants and trees, to be at peace for a few precious moments. No matter how much we may love city life, we also need the nurture of the living Earth.

If you have a garden, you could create a fragrant paradise! Instead of growing those enormous scentless roses so beloved of gardeners nowadays, choose an old-fashioned variety such as *Rosa gallica* or *Rosa damascena*, both of which produce the exquisite essence of rose. Other fragrant plants suitable for most gardens, at least in Britain, include summer-flowering jasmine, phlox, tobacco plants, night-scented stock, ten-week stocks, sweet peas, mignonette, and of course, herbs such as lavender, camomile, rosemary, lemon balm and the many varieties of mint. Narcissus, bluebells, hyacinth and lily-of-the-valley provide scent in the spring, whereas aromatic shrubs such as the flowering currant (also known as ribes), and evergreen trees such as pine and cypress smell wonderful all year round.

As with the blending of essential oils, you can allow yourself to become totally immersed in the act of creative planting, harmonizing scents and colours with the music of nature. Remember that you too are a part of the garden, and in accord with the spirit of the place.

If you do not have a garden, you may be able to grow some fragrant indoor plants. All you need is a sunny window sill and enthusiasm. Jasmine reigns supreme; it can fill a room with the intense fragrance of its white, star-shaped flowers. Other aromatic plants suitable for growing indoors include lemon geranium and the scented leaved pelargoniums, brunfelsia (an evergreen shrub with large fragrant flowers), heliotrope and the lovely gardenia. Though difficult to grow, the gardenia can be a delight indoors. In spring, when the large, waxy, white flowers appear, the surrounding air is filled with fragrance. More simply, you can plant bulbs of hyacinth in the autumn, to bloom in early spring. Their sweet heady scent is reminiscent of both jasmine and jonquil.

This is living, breathing aromatherapy — ambience in the growing!

9 · Other Dimensions

For some time I practised aromatherapy 'by the book', prescribing certain essences for this state of mind or that in accordance with aromatherapy lore, yet at the same time wondering why, for the most part, people did not respond as expected. True, the oils usually had a positive effect, but not in any specific way. Frankincense revealed few new paths, clary sage rarely engendered euphoria and patchouli seduced few into ecstasy!

As we have already seen, the *general* effect on the central nervous system of inhaling different essential oils can be measured by an EEG machine. If the aroma is liked, neroli will have a calming effect, for example, while peppermint will clear the head and act as a mental stimulant. But the *emotional* response, the feelings, memories or images an aroma may evoke (or dispel) are totally subjective and therefore unpredictable. Yet still we hear that rose will cure our jealousy, sandalwood our guilt and orange our self-consciousness.

At the risk of adding further to the myth and magic of aromatherapy, I put forward the notion that it is possible to glean something about the personality and/or present state of mind of an individual not only from their aromatic signature (refer back to the experiment in Chapter 6), but also from the overall pattern of the way they construct their own blends. A more accurate picture can be obtained if the person actually knows nothing of the theory of blending, so that their choice of oils is purely instinctive.

The essential oils which are regarded as top notes (basil, bergamot and peppermint, for example) represent the mental sphere. Essences from the middle range (clary sage, marjoram, rose) are in harmony with the 'heart centre', the feeling, humanitarian aspect of our being, while oils which resonate from the base (patchouli, sandalwood, vetiver) are in tune with the material or physical level. So where a blend displays a disconnection between any of the spheres, it could be said that the person lacks energy in the corresponding area of the mindbody. Should a blend be composed entirely of head and base notes, for example, it would indicate that the composer lacks energy in the heart centre — while such a person may be sensible, practical and down-to-earth, they may also come over as somewhat detached.

To take an example from life: what do you think the following blend says about the composer? (Oils are listed in the order of top, middle, base.)

bergamot
grapefruit
lavender
geranium

As you can see, the blend is composed mainly of top notes, with lavender and geranium forming the heart — but there are no base notes, nor even an oil which resonates from middle to base, which would have compensated somewhat for this lack. This young woman is highly intelligent and in touch with her feelings from both a personal and an humanitarian level. However, the absence of base notes indicates that she is 'ungrounded'. She is rather volatile, possibly prone to nervous tension and is somewhat unworldly. In fact, she is a recently qualified teacher, idealistic with a strong social conscience. However, she finds it extremely difficult to control her often unruly pupils, thus she lies awake at night fretting, wondering whether she should give up teaching.

To take another example, here we have a very different picture:

cypress
cedarwood
patchouli

There are no top notes, which means this person is very much grounded in the here and now. He is not given to flights of fancy, nor does he suffer from mental congestion. Cypress is the highest note, resonating from middle to base, so he is in touch with his feelings; cedarwood confirms this because it resonates from the base to the middle. The deeply resonating patchouli indicates a down-to-earth, yet warm nature. In fact, the composer of this earthy blend (which he uses as a room perfume) is a quiet man in his mid-thirties, a person who is at ease with himself, a physical, kindly soul who loves the great outdoors — hill and mountain walking, and camping in the wilds.

However, we must be very careful not to jump to any rigid conclusions. Just like traditional aromatherapy, the intuitive approach demands a great deal of practice before it can be perfected. Much more needs to be taken into account, not least, the passing physical and emotional state of the composer as reflected in the aromatic signature. Does the aroma smell happy, sad, or in any way harsh or flat? Does it exude a robust quality or is it somewhat delicate and 'colourless'? It is worth remembering that the most difficult feat for the intuitive aromatherapist to master is detachment — it is all too easy to interpret someone else's aromatic signature through the haze of our own subjective responses.

As a matter of interest, the late Marguerite Maury — the founder of holistic aromatherapy — believed strongly in the 'Individual Prescription'. Oils were blended to reflect the person as a whole: mind, body and psyche. When massaged into the skin, the essences were found to be a 'rehabilitator and a restorer of balance'. It was also discovered that aromatherapy enhanced the efficacy of other treatments such as homoeopathy, diet and herbs. As the person's physical and emotional state improved, the Individual Prescription would be changed accordingly. For example, a deeply resonating oil such as sandalwood would be added to a blend displaying a disconnection between the heart and the material level. A top note such as bergamot would embrace the mind of one whose Individual Prescription revealed a disconnection between the heart and the mental sphere. And rose oil (a heart or middle note) would bridge both the mental and material spheres.

Marguerite Maury does not mention in her writings the part aroma preference may have played — her Individual Prescriptions were arrived at mainly by means of crystal-lography and blood spectrography. After all, she was a biochemist. Nevertheless, I am convinced that the simpler aroma preference route gives us a very interesting and fairly accurate guide to the pattern of the mindbody.

Having used your personalized blend for a period of time, say about a month, you may discover that your aroma preference has altered, that you are instinctively drawn to a different oil — an oil that bridges the gap (if you have one)! However, if this does not occur naturally for you, try adding a tiny amount of a 'missing link' essence to the blend (so tiny as to be barely perceptible), gradually increasing the quantity over a period until you discover that its presence has become a wonderful addition to the blend.

There is another way to personalize the effects of essential oils: you can employ the Bach Flower Remedies which, like the homoeopathic 'mentals', are prescribed according to the personality and/or emotional state of the sufferer rather than the physical symptoms of illness. Let us take a look at this intriguing system of healing. It is an approach calling for no medical training, simply a natural sensitivity and feeling for others.

The Bach Flower Remedies

In 1930 a talented physician and homoeopath, Dr Edward Bach, suddenly turned his back on his lucrative London practice to begin a quest which was to change his life. Much to the bewilderment of his medical colleagues, Bach was inspired (for there is no other word for it) to seek a completely new form of medicine, a totally benign method which would harm neither people nor animals. Moreover, he became convinced that poisonous substances of animal, plant or mineral origin should play no part in healing — even when used in infinitesimal doses as in homoeopathy.

Already he had discovered that long continued stress resulting from emotions such as anger, fear or worry lowered a person's resistance to disease. The body would then become prey to all manner of infection or illness, whether it be a cold, shingles, a digestive upset or something much more serious. Moreover, his homoeopathic background had led to the realization that people suffering from the same disease yet sharing similar personalities responded well to a particular remedy, but that others of a different temperament needed other treatment for the same physical complaint. Thus Bach's axiom became: 'Take no notice of the disease, think only of the personality of the one in distress.' Bach also believed that disease is largely the result of emotional disharmony. Moreover, he felt that the key to true healing, healing of body, mind and spirit, lay in the plant kingdom, not in the laboratory. He also sensed that these special healing plants would be found growing wild, nurtured by the living Earth and energized by the synergy of fresh air, rain water and sunlight.

Immediately after leaving London, Bach settled down in a village near Betws-y-coed in North Wales. Living close to nature, his innate sensitivity blossomed fully. Indeed, his sensitivity became so highly developed that he had merely to place a petal on his tongue or hold his hand over a flowering plant to be aware of its effects on the mind and body. Later he was to gain his knowledge in a different way: for some days before the discovery of a healing flower (he felt that the plant's subtle powers were concentrated in the flower rather than in other parts) he experienced in himself the distressing state of mind for which that particular flower was a remedy. Indeed, he suffered intensely in his quest, both physically and mentally.

A Simple Method of Potentization

Bach set out to discover a simple method for capturing the flower energies. At first he prepared the Remedies homoeopathically, but he wanted to develop a much simpler method which would enable most people to prepare the Remedies for themselves, should they so wish.

In fact, he devised two methods of *potentization*, as he called it: the 'Sun Method' and the 'Boiling Method'. In the former, which is the simplest, the best flower heads are carefully picked and put in a thin glass bowl full of springwater. The bowl is then placed in strong sunlight for a few hours, until the energy of the blooms is transferred to the water. Afterwards, the vitalized water or 'essence' is poured into bottles half-filled with brandy, which acts as a preservative. Certain plants, such as Star of Bethlehem, willow and elm, he later decided needed a stronger method of extraction, so he devised the Boiling Method. Here plant material is simmered in water for half an hour before being preserved in brandy. The resulting 'Mother Tincture' from either method of potentization is diluted in a further quantity of brandy and labelled 'Stock'. Although the Stock is a dilution of the original tincture, it is nevertheless considered to be a concentrated remedy because it requires further dilution in water before administration.

Of the 38 Bach Flower Remedies, two are a little different because they are not prepared from wild flowers. These are Rock Water (simply potentized springwater) and Cerato, which is a cultivated plant native to the Himalayas.

How Do They Work?

The Flower Remedies act to transmute negative emotions such as fear, melancholy and hatred into courage, joy and love, and in so doing they are believed to correct the *cause* of our ills. The Flower Remedies do not simply buffer the effects of a turbulent perception, as is the case of some mind-bending substances. Instead, they act as a gentle catalyst, generating change from within.

Just how they achieve this, no one really knows for certain. Their mode of action may be similar to other vibrational healing methods such as colour healing, gem therapy and homoeopathy (refer back to page 19).

Flower Remedies in Practice

The Flower Remedies are a wonderful adjunct to all other forms of treatment, be it orthodox, homoeopathic, herbal or whatever. They work on the mental/spiritual level and will not interfere with any other means of healing the body — in fact, they enhance other forms of treatment.

When used in conjunction with aromatherapy massage, the Flower Remedies help to release ingrained fear and tension, which often manifest as cold, painful, or over-sensitive areas in the body — the feet, solar plexus, shoulders or buttocks, for example. The Remedies appear to hasten the healing process, especially in those who find it extremely difficult to let go.

It has to be emphasized that the Remedies' effect is subtle. They work slowly over a period of say a month or many months, depending on how deep-rooted the distress may be. In the beginning, the Flower energies may only embrace the superficial emotions rather than the deep-rooted fears and conflicts which may be causing the present physical and emotional condition. Slowly but surely, however, one's mental outlook becomes much more positive and optimistic.

Holly, for instance, is the remedy for those who harbour hatred, envy or suspicion. A course of Holly (however long that may take) will enable such a person to give without wanting anything in return and to rejoice, rather than rage, when their friends experience good fortune. Or there is the Vine type: domineering, inflexible and sometimes ruthlessly ambitious. A course of Vine will bring out the positive side of such a personality as seen in the strong but loving leader, a person who can inspire others.

Of course, we all need a dose of Holly or Vine from time to time, when jealousy, greed, anger or bossiness come to the fore. So the Remedies can also be used for temporary negative states of mind. They help to transmute the negativity before it has time to develop into a physical ailment.

143

The most useful and best known of the Remedies is Rescue Remedy, which is a composite of 5 of the 38 Flowers. As its name suggests, it is the Remedy for all emergencies — when there is panic, shock, hysteria, mental numbness, even unconsciousness. Although the Remedy cannot replace medical attention, it can alleviate much of the person's distress whilst awaiting the arrival of medical aid, thus enabling the mind-body's healing processes to commence without delay.

Rescue Remedy is also most helpful in other traumatic situations such as visiting the dentist, receiving bad news, attending court proceedings, etc. It is also helpful when a child is distressed after seeing horror or violence on television.

Bach advised that we should carry a small bottle of Rescue Remedy with us at all times. It is also a good idea to keep a bottle in the bathroom cabinet or in the first aid box.

The five flowers which comprise the Rescue Remedy are:

Star of Bethlehem: for shock and numbness.
Rock Rose: for terror and panic.
Impatiens: for great agitation, irritability and tension.
Cherry Plum: for violent outbursts and hysteria.
Clematis: for the bemused, faraway sensation that often precedes a faint.

Prescribing

Prescribing for others is quite simple if you have a caring, perceptive nature, combined with a broad experience of life. Prescribing for yourself, however, takes a great deal of self-knowledge and honesty. Moreover, it is much more difficult to be objective about yourself when feeling down-hearted. So it may be best to ask a friend, partner or close relative to help you choose the correct Remedy or combination of Remedies (a mixture is often required). But be prepared for a few home truths!

It should not be too difficult to limit your choice to within four Remedies, but if you feel you need five or six, it is better to include them all than unintentionally to omit one of the essential Flowers. You cannot overdose, the Remedies are totally benign and can be taken by people of all ages. However, Bach discovered that the energy of one or two carefully chosen essences was far more effective than the energies of several taken at the same time; a phenomenon also recognized in traditional homoeopathy.

The following reference should serve as a guide to the main negative states of mind for which the Flower Remedies are usually prescribed. However, should you wish to take Bach Flower therapy seriously, much more information about the Remedies is required. Therefore I suggest you obtain one of the excellent books on the subject recommended in the Bibliography.

To round out the picture, also included here are the essential oils most commonly associated with similar emotional states. However, as mentioned earlier, I am not sure we can be very specific about the emotional influence of essential oils — and at the same time, I accept that I may have grasped only a fragment of the whole picture.

The 38 Healers

Agrimony: For inner torture hidden behind a happy-go-lucky façade.
Essential Oils: Bergamot, camomile, geranium, lavender.

Aspen: For inexplicable fears stemming from the psyche, nightmares, fear of some impending evil — that something lurks in the shadows.
Essential Oils: Frankincense, juniper, lavender, rose otto, vetiver.

Beech: For intolerance, criticism and arrogance.
Essential Oils: Geranium, lavender, orange.

Centaury: For those who become willing slaves, lacking the will-power to refuse the demands of others.
Essential Oil: Juniper, rosemary.

Cerato: For those who doubt their own judgement and overly seek the advice of others, those who are often influenced and misguided.
Essential Oils: Cajuput, cardomom, grapefruit, rosemary.

145

Cherry Plum: For those who fear they are losing their mind; for uncontrolled outbreaks of anger or violence.
Essential Oils: Camomile, frankincense, juniper, lavender, marjoram, melissa, neroli, rose otto, sandalwood, vetiver, ylang ylang.

Chestnut Bud: For those who never learn by experience and continually repeat the same mistakes.
Essential Oils: Frankincense, juniper, rosemary.

Chicory: For over-possessiveness, attention-seeking and self-pity.
Essential Oil: Rose otto.

Clematis: For indifference, inattentiveness, dreaminess and absent-mindedness, a need to escape from reality.
Essential Oils: Ginger, juniper, patchouli, rosemary, vetiver.

Crab Apple: For those who feel unclean in body or mind, for self-disgust, overemphasis on trivial detail.
Essential Oil: Juniper.

Elm: For those who feel overcome by responsibility or inadequacy, although normally very capable.
Essential Oils: Bergamot, clary sage, lavender, lemongrass, marjoram, neroli.

Gentian: For those who are easily discouraged — that 'one step forward, two steps back' feeling.
Essential Oils: Bay, bergamot, cajuput, grapefruit, lemon, orange, rose otto.

Gorse: For hopelessness and despair — the feeling that nothing more can be done (though can be persuaded to try again).
Essential Oils: Angelica, bergamot, frankincense, neroli, pine, sandalwood.

Heather: For those who are totally obsessed with their own troubles; for poor listeners.
Essential Oils: Rose, sandalwood.

Holly: For those who are envious, jealous, revengeful and suspicious; for the harbouring of hatred.
Essential Oils: Camomile, lavender, marjoram, melissa, rose otto, ylang ylang.

Honeysuckle: For those who suffer nostalgia and regret, who constantly dwell in the past; for homesickness.
Essential Oils: Basil, bergamot, cypress, juniper, rose otto, rosemary.

Hornbeam: For those who feel tired and weary — that 'Monday morning feeling'.
Essential Oils: Basil, bergamot, black pepper, cardomom, cajuput, coriander, cypress, eucalyptus, grapefruit, hyssop, juniper, lemon, lemongrass, peppermint, pine, rosemary.

Impatiens: For impatience and irritability.
Essential Oils: Camomile, clary sage, lavender, marjoram, melissa, neroli, rose otto, sandalwood, ylang ylang.

Larch: For lack of self-confidence, feelings of inferiority, always anticipating failure.
Essential Oils: Bergamot, rose otto, sandalwood, ylang ylang.

Mimulus: For fear of known things, shyness and timidity.
Essential Oils: Juniper, lavender, neroli, rosemary, vetiver.

Mustard: For those who suffer fluctuating cycles of black depression.
Essential Oils: Bergamot, geranium, lavender.

Oak: For those who suffer despondency as a result of obstinate, relentless effort against all odds.
Essential Oils: Clary sage, frankincense, lavender.

Olive: For those who feel completely exhausted, both physically and mentally; for convalescence.
Essential Oils: Bergamot, clary sage, lavender, vetiver.

147

Pine: For those who suffer from guilt and self-reproach, always blaming themselves for the mistakes of others.
Essential Oils: Pine, sandalwood, ylang ylang.

Red Chestnut: For fear and excessive concern for the welfare of others.
Essential Oils: Lavender, neroli, rose otto.

Rock Rose: For an extremely acute state of fear, terror or panic, including panic attacks.
Essential Oils: Lavender, melissa, neroli, rose otto, vetiver.

Rock Water: For those who are hard on themselves; a too rigid self-discipline; repression and self-denial.
Essential Oils: Bergamot, clary sage, rose otto, sandalwood.

Scleranthus: For indecision, uncertainty, vacillation and mood swings.
Essential Oils: Angelica, basil, cajuput, cardomom, cedarwood, geranium, grapefruit, lavender.

Star of Bethlehem: For the effects of bad news or fright following an accident; the long-term effects of shock which may have occurred in the distant past — a car crash, bereavement and so forth.
Essential Oils: Lavender, melissa, neroli, rose otto.

Sweet Chestnut: For extreme mental anguish, the utmost limits of despair and grief, the times when one is unable even to pray.
Essential Oils: Frankincense, lavender, rose otto.

Vervain: For over-enthusiasm, over-effort and strain; fanaticism.
Essential Oils: Bergamot, camomile, clary sage, geranium, lavender.

Vine: For those who are domineering and inflexible, always striving for power, for the ruthlessly ambitious.
Essential Oils: Marjoram, rose otto.

148 **Walnut:** For those who experience difficulties adjusting to change of any nature, e.g. menopause, divorce, teething, the onset of menstruation.
Essential Oils: Camomile, clary sage, cypress, juniper.

Water Violet: For those who are too proud and aloof; for loneliness.
Essential Oils: Melissa, sandalwood.

White Chestnut: For persistent worrying thoughts and mental arguments; for those unable to sleep.
Essential Oils: Camomile, clary sage, frankincense, lavender, neroli, rose otto.

Wild Oat: For those who feel dissatisfied with life because they have yet to find their true vocation; for boredom and frustration.
Essential Oils: Frankincense, lavender, rosemary, sandalwood.

Wild Rose: For those who are totally resigned to their lot, no matter how hard or mundane, for those making little or no effort for improvement.
Essential Oils: Basil, rosemary.

Willow: For those who feel bitter and resentful — the 'poor me' attitude.
Essential Oils: Grapefruit, rose otto.

Rescue Remedy: An all-purpose remedy for cases of trauma, anguish, shock, bereavement and so forth.
Essential Oil: Lavender.

Buying the Flower Remedies

The Remedies come in little dark-glass dropper bottles of modestly priced Stock Concentrate which can be obtained from many health shops, a few chemists or by mail order (see addresses in the Appendix).

DOSAGE

149

You can take two or three drops of the Stock Concentrate directly on the tongue as required: three times a day for problems of a long-term nature, or much more often in acute states of distress such as fear, emotional shock, anger, examination nerves or whatever. You can also put a couple of drops in a small glass of water or fruit juice to be sipped at intervals throughout the day.

However, the most economical way to take the Remedies is to make up a treatment bottle. The standard dilution is 2 drops from each Stock Concentrate to a 30 ml medicine bottle (obtainable from chemists), three-quarters filled with springwater (or tap water that has been boiled then cooled) and topped up with some brandy to preserve the mixture. If a 30 ml size dropper bottle is difficult to obtain, a slightly smaller or larger bottle will suffice. The dosage is four drops of the diluted Remedy three or four times daily, or more often as required.

Important:
With Rescue Remedy (a composite of five Flowers), the dosage is usually doubled to 4 drops, whether taken neat or diluted in springwater. Furthermore, when combined with other Flowers it is considered to be a single Remedy.

Flowers and Oils

The Flower Remedies can be incorporated into any of your aromatic concoctions. Although insoluble in oil (due to the brandy preservative) the quantity required is so tiny that any separation of oil and Flower Remedy is hardly noticeable.

Massage Oils

Add 1 or 2 drops of an appropriate Stock Concentrate to the saucer of oil. Alternatively, add 3 — 4 drops to a 100 ml bottle of massage oil.

Compresses

Bach prescribed compresses in addition to internal doses of the Remedies for cases of external lesions such as skin eruptions and inflammation or sprains and strains.

To make a compress, add 6 drops of Stock Concentrate to a hot or cold aromatic compress as described on page 79.

Suggested Flowers

Crab Apple is commonly used for skin problems such as acne, eczema and psoriasis. It is the only Remedy that is prescribed specifically for a physical ailment. However, it should be combined with oral doses of other Flower Remedies prescribed according to the individual's personality or mood. Crab Apple is especially helpful to those who feel unclean or suffer from feelings of self-disgust because of their skin complaint.

Rescue Remedy is a helpful addition to an aromatic compress for swellings, bruises, sprains and so forth.

Baths

You can add the Flower Remedies to an aromatic bath to augment oral doses of the Remedies and to enhance the effect of the essential oils. Use 5 drops of each chosen Stock Concentrate to the bath water, and 6–8 drops of essential oil.

SUGGESTED BLENDS

For tiredness and exhaustion, especially in convalescence:
Flower Remedies: Hornbeam or Olive.
Essential Oils: If you like the aroma, a blend of clary sage and vetiver is a fortifying combination (e.g. 3 drops of vetiver, 4 drops of clary sage). Other suitable essences include citrus oils, coriander, geranium, rosemary and tea tree.

For nervous tension and 'mental chatter':
Flower Remedies: Rescue Remedy and/or White Chestnut.
Essential Oils: If you like the aroma, a blend of bergamot, clary sage and neroli is a calming combination (e.g. 2 drops of neroli, 2 drops of clary sage, 4 drops of bergamot). Other suitable essences include camomile, cypress, frankincense, juniper, marjoram, rose otto and sandalwood.

Skin and Hair Care

As we have already seen, Crab Apple can be helpful for skin eruptions. Use 2 drops to 100 ml of distilled water, or add the drops to one of the skin tonic recipes suggested in Chapter 6.

Similarly, Crab Apple can be added to anti-dandruff treatments, and also to essential oil preparations for head lice. No matter how often we are told (or how often we tell our children) that there is nothing shameful about catching head lice and that the lice actually prefer clean hair, it is difficult not to feel unclean or to harbour a certain amount of self-disgust when you have head lice. This is where Crab Apple can help, and also Rescue Remedy if the discovery comes as a great shock.

Rescue Remedy is a wonderful addition to the antiseptic ointment recipe on page 103. Add about 4 drops to the melted beeswax and oil mixture. You can also add Rescue (or any other appropriate Flower Remedy) to a bland commercial preparation. Stir in 4 drops to every 30 g of cream or ointment, and 3 drops to 25 ml of lotion.

Although it may sound flippant, how about making a 'No Regrets' skin cream or skin tonic? I remember reading somewhere that the negative emotion of regret accelerates the ageing process of the skin. Therefore Honeysuckle is now the star ingredient of all my skin care concoctions!

No doubt you can think of many other ways of combining Flowers with oils. Do let me know what you discover.

And Finally . . .

A final wish: may you enjoy many timeless moments of creative aromatherapy — of strolling through enchanted woodlands, of breathing the invigorating air of high places, of summer rain and fragrant earth, of sultry nights and roses. And not forgetting those curious moments of fantasia — of feeling, tasting, hearing, seeing fragrance . . . and other dimensions of wonder!

Further Reading

Ackerman, D., *A Natural History of the Senses* (Chapmans, 1990).

Fischer-Rizzi, Susanne, *Complete Aromatherapy Handbook* (Sterling Publishing, New York, 1990).

Hodgkinson, L., *How to Banish Cellulite Forever* (Grafton, 1989).

Kenton, L., *The Joy of Beauty* (Century, 1984).

Maury, M., *Marguerite Maury's Guide to Aromatherapy* (C.W. Daniel, 1989).

Maxwell-Hudson, C., *The Complete Book of Massage* (Dorling Kindersley, 1988).

Scheffer, M., *Bach Flower Therapy: Theory and Practice* (Thorsons, 1984).

Wildwood, C., *Flower Remedies* (Element Books, 1991).

——, *Holistic Aromatherapy* (Thorsons, 1992).

Essential Oil Suppliers

The following suppliers stock a range of high quality aromatherapy grade oils. Kittywake and Bodytreats also stock separately labelled organically produced oils from plants grown without the use of chemical fertilizers and poisonous sprays.

United Kingdom

Bodytreats Ltd
15 Approach Road
Raynes Park
London SW20 8BA

Butterbur & Sage
101 Highgrove Street
Reading
RG1 5EJ

Kittywake Oils
Cae Kitty
Taliaris
Llandeilo
Dyfed
SA19 7DP

United States of America

Aroma Vera Inc.
PO Box 3609
Culver City
California 90231

Neal's Yard USA
284 Connecticut St
San Francisco
California 94107

For essential oils and aromatherapy courses, contact:

United Kingdom

Purple Flame Aromatics
61 Clinton Lane
Kenilworth
Warwickshire
CV8 1AS

United States of America

American AromaTherapy
Association
PO Box 1222
Fair Oaks
California 95628

Australia

Berida Manor
PO Box 350
Bowral
New South Wales 2576

For aromatherapy courses, contact:

The London School of
Aromatherapy
PO Box 780
London NW5 1DY

For a list of accredited aromatherapists, send a stamped addressed envelope
to:

The International Federation of Aromatherapists
The Department of Continuing Education
The Royal Masonic Hospital
London W6 0TN

For cosmetic materials and herbs, contact:

Baldwins
71–3 Walworth Road
London SE17

The following are Bach Flower Remedy suppliers. Please enclose a
stamped addressed envelope with all enquiries:

United Kingdom	*United States of America*
The Bach Centre	Dr Edward Bach Healing Society
Mount Vernon	644 Merrick Road
Sotwell	Lynbrook
Wallingford	New York 11563
Oxon	
OX10 OPZ	

The Flower Remedy Programme
PO Box 65
Hereford
HR2 OUW

Therapeutic Index

abscess 36
acne 30, 31, 34, 36, 39, 42, 43, 88,
   103, 104–5
AIDS 22
allergy 25, 28, 30, 33, 114
anaemia 37
anger 146
anorexia 37, 106
anxiety 30, 31, 32, 33, 35, 36, 37, 39,
   40, 41, 43
appetite, loss of 32
arthritis 35, 37, 40, 41, 79
athlete's foot 36, 39, 40, 43

blood pressure
   high 12, 32, 36, 37, 43
   low 42
boils 29, 30, 32, 36
breastfeeding 34
bronchitis 28, 31, 33, 34, 36, 37, 38,
   39, 40, 41, 42
bruises 37
burns 33, 36, 41

catarrh 31, 33, 34, 38, 40, 42
cellulite 29, 33, 34, 35, 37, 39, 92–3
chilblains 30, 35, 36, 37
cholesterol, high 41
circulation, poor 30
cold sores 29, 30, 33, 37, 39, 40, 41,
   43
colds 28, 33, 35, 36, 37
colic 30, 32
colitis 30
constipation 30, 37
convalescence 147
convulsions 42
coughs 28, 30, 31, 33, 34, 35, 36, 38,
   40, 42, 43
criticism 145
cystitis 29, 30, 33, 35, 36, 40, 42

dandruff 30, 36, 39, 41, 43, 101, 152

depression 29, 31, 32, 36, 38, 39, 41,
   42, 43
diabetes 33, 34
diarrhoea 33, 38, 42

eczema 27, 30, 31, 35, 36, 147, 151

fainting 36, 40
fear 143, 145, 146, 148
fever 29, 33, 39
fibrositis 96
flatulence 36, 37, 38
'flu 30, 33, 37, 40, 41, 43
fluid retention 34, 35, 37, 39

gallstones 37
gargle 35
gout 35
grief 148
gums, disorders of 32, 33, 38, 102

haemorrhoids 33, 34, 35, 38
hair
   falling 41
   growth, to stimulate 102
   thinning 39
   treatments for 93–4, 101
hangover 41
hayfever 33
hayfever balm, recipe for 99
head lice 36, 40, 41, 94, 152
headache 28, 37, 41
hysteria 38, 43

incontinence 33
indigestion 30, 37, 40, 41
irritability 147
insect stings 32, 36, 37, 43
insomnia 30, 32, 36, 38, 40, 42, 43
intolerance 145

joints, inflammation of 30

lethargy 34, 40
leucorrhoea 32, 33, 36, 37, 41

measles 33
menopause 30, 33, 41, 148
menstruation
  absence of 31, 35, 38
  heavy 33, 41
  irregular 41
  painful 32, 33, 36
  scanty 28, 36
mental fatigue 28, 41, 124
migraine 30, 33, 36, 37, 40, 42
mood swings 36, 148
mouth ulcers 34, 38
muscular pain 30, 35, 36, 37, 43, 91

nausea 40
nervous debility 32, 42
nervous tension 33, 35, 36, 37, 38,
    40, 42, 43, 44, 151
neuralgia 30, 33, 34

palpitations 38, 40, 42, 44
panic attacks 12
perspiration, excessive 32, 33
pre-menstrual syndrome (PMS) 29,
    31, 32, 35, 36, 37, 38, 40, 42
psoriasis 30, 151

rheumatism 30, 32, 33, 35, 37, 40, 92
ringworm 34, 43

scabies 40
scarlet fever 33
sciatica 96
shingles 34

shock, emotional 38, 43, 148, 149
sinusitis 28, 33, 40, 124
skin, care of 68—73
  ageing 34, 38, 41, 45, 90
  cracked 39
  dry 39, 89
  inflamed 79, 81, 89, 96
  oily 32, 33, 35, 42, 103
sensitive 28, 90
skin cancer 94
skin pigmentation 29, 37, 39
skin ulcers 33, 38
sores 39
sprains 30, 33, 36
stomach pain 30
stress 32, 45—46
stretch marks 98
swellings 30

teeth 102
thread veins 30, 33, 41
throat, infections of 32, 33, 34, 35,
    36, 37, 40, 42
thrush 34, 38, 43
tiredness 147
tonsilitis 29
toothache 32

uterine disorders 41

varicose veins 33
veruccae 37, 43
voice, loss of 33

warts 37, 43
whooping cough 32
wounds 30, 33, 34, 37, 38, 40, 42, 43

General Index

absolutes 20—1
aftershave 101
angelica 111, 112, 131, 146, 148
anosmia 14
antibiotics 31, 39, 40
antiseptics 33
anti-virals 22, 31
aphrodisiacs 22, 32, 35, 38, 39, 41, 42,
   43, 133
aroma
   emotion and 12, 22, 137
   memory and 9—10
   preference 14, 15, 22, 27, 77, 106—7,
     140
   stereochemical theory of 13
   vibration and 17—8
aromatic signature 18, 86—7, 139
aromatic water 109, 119—20
attunement 107—8
avocado oil 80
Aztecs 133

babies 27
baby oil 79
Bach, Edward 15, 140—1
Bach Remedies 16, 81, 140—52
base oils 79—80, 89
basil 28, 111, 112, 115, 124, 127, 147,
   148
baths 73, 151
bay 146
beeswax 81
Benveniste, Jacques 16
bergamot 29, 78, 91, 111, 117, 118,
   120, 123, 124, 127, 129, 130, 131,
   145, 146, 147
black pepper 29—30, 92, 112, 115,
   127, 147
blending 106—7
borax 96
Brewer's yeast 81, 103

cajuput 145, 146, 147, 148

calendula oil 89, 95
camomile 30, 89, 90, 93, 95, 101, 115,
   116, 145, 146, 147, 149, 151
cardomom 112, 115, 118, 127, 145,
   147, 148
cedarwood 30—1, 91, 92, 101, 112,
   117, 118, 129, 132, 148
children 27
China 11
chocolate 133—4
cider vinegar 82, 100
cinnamon bark 31, 78, 112, 115, 127,
   129
clary sage 31—2, 91, 117, 118, 128,
   130, 146, 147, 148, .151
clove 32, 78, 112, 115, 129
cocoa butter 81, 98
coconut oil 81
cologne 109, 111, 120
compress 74—5, 150—1
   facial 70
coriander 32—3, 108, 111, 120, 124,
   127, 130, 147, 151
cypress 33, 88, 118, 123, 127, 147,
   148, 151

distillation 20

eau de cologne 111, 120
Egyptians 10—11
essential oils 15, 19—26, 27—44, 75
   caring for 25—6
   chemistry 24
   definition of 19
   effects on mind 15
   extraction methods 20—1
   properties of 21—4
   skin absorption 23
ethyl alcohol 109
eucalyptus 33—4, 94, 95, 111, 115,
   127, 147
evening primrose oil 89, 90
exfoliation 72—3

face packs 71, 104—5
feathering 65—6
fennel 103, 111, 112, 115
footbath 73—4
frankincense 11, 34, 115, 117, 118, 128, 132, 145, 146, 147, 148, 149
Fuller's Earth 81
fumigants 31, 32, 76

garlic oil 23
geranium 34—5, 88, 93, 94, 103, 112, 117, 129, 130, 135, 145, 147, 148
ginger 35, 115, 118, 127, 131, 146
glycerin 96—7
grapefruit 111, 117, 120, 123, 127, 131, 145, 146, 147, 148
grapeseed oil 80

homoeopathy 16
honey 82, 103, 105
hormones 22
hypericum oil 89, 95
hyssop 11

jasmine 20
jojoba 80
juniper 35—6, 118, 124, 127, 131, 132, 145, 146, 147

lactic acid 103
lavender 36, 88, 89, 91, 93, 94, 95, 98, 101, 104, 117, 118, 120, 123, 126, 127, 128, 129, 130, 132, 145, 146, 147, 148
lemon 36—7, 111, 118, 127, 146
lemon balm 95
lemongrass 111, 112, 115, 146, 147
lime 92, 111, 117, 118, 120, 127
lip salve, recipe for 100

mandarin 92, 111, 127, 129
marigold oil 95
marjoram 37, 91, 146, 147, 148
massage 46—67
massage oil 49, 68—9, 88—90, 150
  mixing of 84—6
Maury, Marguerite 139—40
meditation 34
melissa 146, 147, 148, 149
mind, nature of 16—7
mineral oil; see baby oil
moisturisers 96—7
mouthwash, recipe for 102
myrrh 37—8, 77, 90, 102, 112, 115

neroli 38, 78, 98, 117, 118, 120, 129, 146, 147, 148, 151
neurochemicals 16—7

oatmeal 103
odour intensity 115
ointment, recipe for 98
olive oil, extra virgin 79
orange 38—9, 92, 111, 118, 120, 127
orange flower water 98
organic oils 21

palma rosa 112
patchouli 39, 88, 91, 92, 93, 102, 112, 114, 117, 118, 128, 146
peppermint 39—40, 100, 102, 111, 115, 117, 118, 147
perfume 76, 108—20
petitgrain 40, 110, 117, 120, 123, 127, 129
pheromones 13
pine 40—1, 100, 112, 118, 123, 127, 146, 147
potentization 141—2

quantum physics 17—8

Rescue Remedy 143—4
room perfumes 31, 75—76, 121—35
rose otto 41, 78, 112, 115, 117, 145, 146, 147, 148, 151
rosemary 41—2, 88, 92, 93, 94, 102, 118, 123, 127, 129, 145, 146, 147, 151
rosewater 98, 130
rosewood 21

sage 95
sandalwood 14, 42, 93, 102, 112, 127, 128, 130, 146, 147, 149
sauna, facial 70—1
skin brushing 71—2
skin cream, recipes for 98
skin tonics, recipes for 100—1
smell, sense of 12—13, 14
smell-testing 113—14
St John's wort oil 95
sunscreens, recipes for 94—5
synergy 23
synthetic oils 24—5

tagetes 112, 115
tea tree 42—3, 88, 94, 95, 99, 103, 111, 151

tuberose 20

valerian 106, 131
Valnet, Jean 22—3
vanilla 112, 133—4
vaporizers 121—2
vegetable oils 79—80
vetiver 43, 91, 112, 117, 128, 130,
    145, 146, 147, 148, 151

vibration 17—8

witch hazel 101

ylang ylang 43—4, 90, 93, 112, 117,
    118, 126, 129, 146, 147
yoghurt 81, 103